DYSPEPSIA AND IBS FOR THE WISE

How to Treat Functional Digestive Disorders (FDDs)

with or without Medication

By
Larry Tremblay

B.A. Philosophy, B.A. Management economics

First English Edition

Back photo by Chantale Tremblay.
Text revision (French version) : Lise Bédard et Amélie Lapierre.
Translation : Amerique traductions – 1192 Rue Du Domaine, Cap-Rouge (QC), G1Y 2E1 – Phone: 418-652-9247.

Edition and distribution:
Larry Tremblay, Editor. 2518, chemin du Foulon, Québec (Qc), Canada G1T 1X7 (tremblay.larry@videotron.ca)

Avis to librarians: this book is in the catalogue of Library and Archives Canada: (www.collectionscanada.ca/amicus/index-f.html)
Preceding French editions: ISBN 1-4251-1432-6 and ISBN: 2-9806102-1-2
Printed at Victoria, BC, Canada.
Canada, United States, Ireland, England

Order this book online at www.trafford.com
or email orders@trafford.com

Most Trafford titles are also available at major online book retailers.

Print information available on the last page.

ISBN: 978-1-4269-8868-4 (sc)
ISBN: 978-1-4269-8963-6 (e)

Trafford rev. 03/02/2015

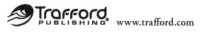 www.trafford.com

North America & international
toll-free: 1 888 232 4444 (USA & Canada)
fax: 812 355 4082

CONTENTS

THANKS

I would like to thank Chantale Tremblay, my wife who, sometimes at the risk of hurting my pride, gave me the chance of knowing and taking better care of myself. I would also like to thank Normand, my son, to whom I provided my care, who did not question it, and who gave me the joy of seeing him suffer less than I did at his age.

I also thank my collaborators for the first edition of the work: Francine Allard, Jocelyne Raymond and Dave Tremblay (revision), André Dion for his sound advices, Lise Bédard (secretaryship), as well as Sigrid Choquette, for the pre-edition.

I particularly wish to emphasize the generous contribution of Dr Pierre Poitras, gastroenterologist, who commented the second and third editions, and who supported me in this journey.

I would like to thank readers of my first editions, especially those who forwarded their comments which gave me the courage to go on with my works.

Finally, I would like to thank the *Journal* (*Association des employées et des employés du gouvernement du Québec*), the *Journal Vert* and *Du Cœur au ventre*, the *Association des maladies gastro-intestinales fonctionelles* (AMGIF) review who published some of my works on functional digestive disorders, and *Le Devoir*, *Le Soleil* and *Canoe. ca* who published an article on my book.

PREFACE TO THE THIRD EDITION

Compared with the first two editions, this one includes a literature review. It basically completes the writings I undertook more than a decade ago. The "Literature Review" section deals both with the identification and with the pharmacological treatments of most of the symptoms already dealt with in the "Personal Approach" section. It also describes a few original approaches, such as those proposed by Pierre Pallardy and Drs Servan-Schreiber and Devroede.

The "Literature Review" section is divided into six parts: the Rome Diagnostic Criteria, meant as an international recognition of the diagnosis, terminology and treatments related to functional digestive disorders (FDDs); the description and treatments recommended for the most common ailments (flatulence, reflux, constipation, diarrhea, migraine, etc.); a few known causes of abdominal pain (food, allergies, diseases, etc.); some recent hypotheses (central nervous system, traumas, psychosomatic causes, depression); exercise suggestions from some authors; and, recommended means of alleviating some of the symptoms (homeopathy, herbal medicine, diet, food supplements).

Although the book deals with what can be done naturally to ease symptoms related to FDDs, the bulk of the information compiled in the literature review is about medical care and the medical conditions requiring the advice of a health care practitioner. To care for ourselves properly we need the best information possible, to decide when to turn to medical science or to other health care methods. This information should also help us prepare for our visit to the health care professional. Since FDDs are known to have a strong psychosomatic component, many doctors find that patients with this complaint are difficult to treat. When a patient is fairly well-informed, he or she can have a better relationship with his or her doctor, a fact recognized as one of the conditions for effective medical care.

Some criteria prevailed in the writing of the "Literature Review." I tried to exclude promotional information as much as possible. I also tried to leave out any information that is unproven or scientifically weak. For example, in this edition I left out an article on *Candida albicans* on the suggestion of Dr Pierre Poitras, gastroenterologist, since the claims made by the author in a book written on the subject have been invalidated by research. However, I retained the information I found interesting, even though it was not entirely proven. This information is found mainly at the end of chapter four and also in chapter five. It is handled in a more editorial fashion. My goal is to inform, but also to appeal to the reader's judgment. There are people who look for magic formulas, sometimes insistently, to ease their discomfort. Like medical doctors I do not believe in miracle cures to treat FDDs, but this doesn't mean that a little curiosity is wrong.

According to Dr Michael Oppenheim, biofeedback and antidepressants share similar effects in alleviating FDDs, although biofeedback is more costly in terms of learning, and more difficult to apply. However, in my opinion, whatever the approach, the results will be improved if the gas release and relaxation techniques are used in combination with it. I am convinced that FDD-related symptoms can often be treated effectively through continuing efforts, a generous and caring attitude towards oneself, better self-knowledge and... good judgment (hence the title *Dyspepsia and IBS for the Wise*).

Finally, because FDDs are often linked to child abuse, post-traumatic stress syndrome, long-term effects of operations or gastrointestinal problems experienced abroad, this book is intended as a work of compassion. Several readers told me about their pain. Many times they did not take good care of themselves, if only to appear normal. They often mentioned that my expertise and the recommended exercises, finally "permitted", greatly helped to set them free. I hope this edition will confirm the importance of taking good care of ourselves, like the child we used to be needed to be treated: with gentleness, patience, perseverance and hope, but also and most of all, with "movements".

Quebec, January 10, 2006.

1 – INTRODUCTION

I am not a doctor. I have been suffering from dyspepsia and from the irritable bowel syndrome (IBS) since my earliest days. I experimented with several approaches and tried to develop the ones that best applied to me, sometimes on the spur of the moment. My approach is meant to complement the medical one. The sensitivity and perseverance this approach requires are not obvious and are not taught. However, I can assure you that they allowed me to control my symptoms, even if they sometimes seemed to be sailing on an unpredictable, cruel and all-consuming sea.

The "Personal Approach" section describes in simple terms the symptoms I experienced, as well as some of the hypotheses I developed to understand and in order to relieve FDDs. This should help readers find their way and understand my approach. I then explain in detail the exercises for gas evacuation and for the release of nervous tension, and consequently, of pain. As this is a little known approach, as far as I know, I explain in detail the exercises and the various levels of improvement one can expect.

The spirit in which I approached this book is strangely similar to that of Peter Pan, the mythical symbol of my own generation (*baby-boomers*). When we were young, we all experienced a feeling of intense energy that could help us get well, play outside and run. I can still recall such moments, one could say, moments touched by grace when I felt that my energy would let me overcome all the potential trials and tribulations of life. Unfortunately, as time goes by and even more so for someone suffering from FDDs, we tend to forget this feeling of total energy. We begin to think that we will never feel it again. On the contrary, like Peter Pan, we should never stop believing and... try our best to achieve it. Moreover, we should transcend our pain and overcome the feeling of failure and despondency. We have to keep going, experiment, and move. What would Peter Pan be like if he hadn't fought Captain Hook? And what if he was, in fact, this pain, physical as well as psychological, that assails and paralyses us? And what if he was memory and the fear of those who hurt us? If, as mentioned by Dr Daniel Dufour in his book *Les tremblements intérieurs* (p. 24), illness "only conveys the message of a deep or superficial error in people's attitude towards life". As sports enthusiasts will say: "Triumph without peril brings no glory." Well, today, at fifty four, I am much happier, more optimistic, less unwell, and I am much more involved in sports than I was at thirty. I experience once again the wonderful energy I felt when I was a child. How I wish you felt the same!

As mentioned by Dr Scott Peck, the psychiatrist, in his book *People of the lie* (p. 44): "Healing is the result of love. It is a function of love. Wherever there is love there is healing. And wherever there is no love there is precious little–if any–healing. Paradoxically, a psychology of evil must be a loving psychology. It must be brimful of the love of live. Every step of the way its methodology must be submitted not only to the love of truth but also to the love of life: of warmth and light and laughter, and spontaneity and joy, and service and human caring." If you substitute the symptoms and pain related to FDDs to Dr Peck's psychology of evil, you will understand the purpose of this work: the knowledge and treatment of the symptoms to achieve a good life. I hope this book will mean, for you, as for Peter Pan, the start of a fascinating journey that will help you recover the joy of life.

I was introduced to the release of gases by my wife who, like me, is a long-time dyspepsia sufferer, without knowing it. It was during her pregnancy that she discovered the benefits of releasing gas from the stomach. The regular release of gas saved us from many sleepless nights and much discomfort. We have a twenty year old son who showed me, when he was still small and I was experimenting with the gas release exercises, that babies weren't the only ones who needed to "burp."

Some will tell you that there is no cure for FDDs. Like Peter Pan, I dream that I am cured, it is my challenge! Without being completely cured, with the help of regular exercises, I live my life as if I was, because at the earliest sign of pain or symptoms I do the exercises to help eliminate them. I hope my experience will enable as many of you as possible to get some relief from FDDs.

2 – My Story

There is a theory (see the section on the book written by Dr Devroede) which suggests that the irritable bowel syndrome (IBS) is often the result of the quality of the care provided in early childhood. Learning how to take care of a child depends as much on the parents' personality as on the way they learned to care for others and for themselves. Therefore, we can presume that digestive problems are passed on from one generation to the next. In these pages, I describe my own history and that of my family.

My "problems" began at my birth. According to my mother I suffered from unending colic, sometimes accompanied by fever. She said that I had taught her "sleepless nights". To get me to sleep, she had me lay on her side her and rocked me. After six months of this regimen she let me cry alone in my bed for three nights: her problem was solved; but my digestive problems persisted. Occasionally I had acute indigestion accompanied by faintness.

I suffered from anxiety and insomnia. I numbed the pain by rocking and singing to myself throughout the night, like a caged animal—to the great displeasure of my parents—to compensate for my mother's reassuring presence during my first six months of life. The result was that I had a room all to myself since my older brother couldn't stand me. I ended up by loosening up... out of sheer exhaustion. As fear gave me abdominal pain, so the abdominal pain fed the fear!

My mother had opened a business on the year of my birth. She was very active and didn't have time to take care of us. She had hired a maid. Between the ages of one and three I did not let her hold me in her arms. The only way to get me to calm down was to put me in a child's bed, isolated in what we used to call a "furnace room." Ours had a window through which I could see the children playing outside. Day or night, when I suffered from insomnia, I was in the habit of holding in my stools and my urine for as long as I could. The movement of the stools, and especially the gases, was for me a major source of entertainment, and the only way I could postpone the care!

During the course of my psychoanalysis I recalled that my mother would change my diaper in the evening and at night, when nobody else would do it. My father had two jobs, including one that kept him busy until the middle of the night. When she took care of me my mother pricked me repeatedly with the diaper pins. This made me howl and, paradoxically, it made her laugh. Naturally, she comforted me afterwards. She would then say: "Me and my left hand!" When I was about two and a half, during a diaper change, I became aware of this little game. I began to cry and she took me in her arms. This is when I saw my father, an uncle and my brother seated at the table in the dining room. I started crying even more strongly to "rouse" them so that they would come and protect me from my mother. Nobody reacted. So I told myself that I could never count on them in the future, and that I would be alone to face life with mother … my night mother. When she put me back on the countertop to finish changing me, I made a promise to myself that, some day, I would pull out these pricks from my body. A child promise that I had forgotten, naturally.

Before discovering this little game I had been having strong intermittent pain that "cut through the skin" as if a hair was being pulled out of my abdomen, or a sting came out of my stomach or my legs. It was by analysing this phenomenon that I managed to remember the promise I had made to myself. It was as if the pricks were coming out of my body, one at a time. It was right then that

I became aware that I was on the road to recovery, me and my sometimes "stinging" remarks! Since I had younger brothers and sisters, I remembered that they had also been pricked regularly. To them, at the time, I was one of those "you can't count on". During a discussion with my youngest brother, he told me that he also recalled having been pricked and that, unlike me who had put "this" in my abdomen; he had put it in his head.

My mother's behaviour also had its counterpart in language. She was in the habit of saying things that always made me go out of my mind. Instead of getting angry I became paralysed, as if in shock or waiting to be able to "digest" her words. I realized that my first reaction to inhibited anger was a strong contraction of the large intestine. This caused constipation, and after a few days this invariably caused diarrhea, which was often accompanied by a migraine and a depressed state. When I was older I was often tactless or so awkward that I hurt myself. Instead of rebelling, I recalled my mother's history: in her family, the father regularly beat the children, my mother more often than the others. I thought that she had made us suffer a lot less that what she herself had endured. Should I asked for anything more?

My father also suffered from abdominal pain all his life; he experienced this discomfort as something inevitable, unconscious. He was under the impression that any attempt to change his habits was bound to fail. My mother claims that she always knew him sick. Around the age of thirty he had lost weight and when he was about forty he needed to have surgery for a stomach ulcer but he refused, preferring instead to look after himself and be on the alert for a time. In the night he regularly suffered from indigestion. He developed stomach cancer in 1995 and died a year later, the cancer having spread throughout his body.

He found it difficult to assert himself and often ended up exploding in hysterical fits of anger when he was with relatives or when sensitive issues were discussed (such as religion, sex, money, school, managing the family business, etc.). He would often spark off discussions on these issues, apparently not realizing, we feared, that it would turn sour in the end. He also tended to isolate himself and worked hard manually in order to "forget or not think", as he was found of saying. He was also very idealistic, to the point of rubbing people the wrong way by judging them, looking down on them or telling them what to do. My mother could not resign herself to leaving us alone with him. He would often put us down or miss the mark. My mother would then try to make up for it. In addition, he often hurt himself so that she also had to look after him.

He came from a large family, and most of them died relatively early from cancer. Having served in the military and been at the front in 39-45, he was sometimes very strict on the smallest details but totally overtaken by a relationship of authority. He'd say: "You find what's good for you, I don't know anything about it", which did not prevent him from having opinions about us that were sometimes hard and very firm. My mother believed he was a very sick man. That's why we had to be more reasonable than he was, letting him believe that he was winning, that he was right, that he was the boss!

My mother thought that his "sickness" came from his military experience. Since I have a son and brothers who have learning difficulties, I realized that his problems were mostly related to communication (inflexibility, inability to look people in the eye, anxiety, awkwardness, fear of the unexpected, etc.). My father was especially threatening in situations of communication, when he could become unpredictable, "cutting" and incapable of empathy.

I have a sister who suffers from an incurable disease, who never talked, who could not walk when she was seven and who, at the age of fifty or so, still lives in an institution. My parents wanted at the beginning to take care of it themselves, and keep us out of it. But to be able to manage everything they had to resign themselves to put us in an orphanage, my brother and I, for a few years. My brother, who was there for four years, told me one day that all the kids at the orphanage suffered from chronic constipation, as if they were waiting for their mother to finally let go. I again started the game with my bowels, to the extent that I would often dirty my underwear. I found myself having to wear a diaper for a week, like a few of the children "in detention", and sometimes having to wash my underwear and getting beaten. But we couldn't always ask for permission to go and "do our business" when we were in class. We had to hold it in... and not only for "the fun of it"!

The institution itself seemed to generate a constipation of sorts. To save money, the nuns had us cut pieces of newspapers—eight by twelve centimetres or three by five inches—provided by donors. We weren't allowed to use more than two pieces to wipe ourselves because it clogged up the toilet. This would of course lead to punishments for lack of cleanliness or for clogging up the toilet. I was also often beaten while I learned piano or rehearsing songs and plays. This sums up my experience with my "mothers" of constipation!

Naturally, this got sorted out when I came back home. However, at home they had to resign themselves to putting my sister in an institution. I felt that something had been broken. My father, especially, apparently found it difficult to accept our problems, the demands of us children, especially our illnesses: the only one who was really sick was my sister. Since we were healthy we had better stand up straight (hold it in!) I was the one who had expressed the wish not to go back to the orphanage. Without ever saying it, I always suffered from guilt, from the feeling of having pushed my sister out of the family. I always feared I would be punished for it in the end. I hid behind a kind of arrogance: in response they took pleasure in my difficulties... which I obviously deserved.

It was very difficult for me to communicate with my parents. I wanted to go unnoticed. Both of them, in their own way, were trying to know more about me, but I remained uncommunicative. They knew nothing of my "intestinal" conflicts since I dreaded their "care".

When I grew up, my digestive problems appeared to be under control, but I still suffered from insomnia. However, until the age of 35, about once a year I experienced a period of euphoria when I felt I was in control, that everything was just fine, especially with school or work. This often occurred four days after I visited my parents, or towards the end of the school year. Invariably, after these few days of excitement, I had an acute indigestion with faintness. When I was younger these periods were especially difficult for my father, who was afraid something was not right with my head: Did I suffer from epilepsy like my sister? After I underwent a number of tests the doctors could find nothing wrong with me. It even seemed that I had excellent cerebral functions... probably good enough to become a writer! As I got older, I felt great relief after indigestion, but a little down. Unfortunately, feelings of euphoria, of being competent, were not for me.

I lived for the day when everything would be better. I felt increasingly older, my world was shrinking, even though I wanted the exact opposite; and I couldn't practice sports or concentrate for very long because of my back pain. I had problems with my digestion and regularly suffered from tinnitus (hissing) in my ears and migraines. After I earned my B.A. in Philosophy, I experienced my first bout of depression, followed by a second phase in my early thirties. When I was thirty years old, taking the bus home after work, I asked myself where my life was heading. By logically projecting into the future the way I was feeling then, I came to the conclusion that my horizon was becoming increasingly limited, increasingly dark. Even if I read a lot to entertain myself, to live vicariously, despite my efforts, this vision of a darkening future would not fade.

I stopped reading completely and started psychoanalysis, a promise I had made to myself as a teenager when I was reading Freud and waiting for my life to be brighter, or better, waiting to have something interesting to write about. My older brother had told me I had some good ideas, that I should begin writing. When I was seventeen I answered him that I was more of a consumer of culture than a producer: I was probably already constipated! However, the seed had been sown.

I found it very difficult to complete my studies, especially in management economics. I had to fight my tendency to procrastinate.

I remember that I had to leave aside my fear of success, my sometimes irresistible taste for failure. Because to succeed meant to lay myself open; it meant letting myself be known, be recognized. Whether I was recognized by my parents, by the nuns or by any other authority figure, it meant that I would be "making contact" and so, more or less consciously, taking the risk that people would once again make me suffer. So, what I had to do was to take one session at a time, one course at a time, one day at a time and, to the best of my ability, forget my taste for failure and procrastination, forget success altogether, start anew. However, at the end of almost every session the cycle of acute indigestion, loss of consciousness and depression would begin again.

After entering the job market I had a great deal of difficulty accepting authority. I was prone to frequent fits of anger: the bosses were conspiring against me. I was scared of meeting important people. I also had few friends and could not hold onto them. I constantly had to preserve myself from socially self-destructive behaviors to avoid "engaging in relationships." My migraines were becoming more frequent. When I felt bad, it was undoubtedly somebody's fault!

To suffer, and to feel deep down that my relatives also suffered, to know that I was powerless before all this suffering, prompted me to act. I had hoped that time and some attention would help everything fall into place. However, I soon fell into the hell of good intentions. I could not let us, my family and I, remain in that situation.

Discovering that I could make myself feel better, but not being able to communicate it, although I came across people who really needed it, is a fairly cruel dilemma. I could barely stand to see my father, who just wouldn't listen, plagued with problems that were similar to mine and to be powerless, wordless, to relieve this suffering.

Sometimes, when I was undergoing analysis, I had the feeling that I was running around in circles, especially when my symptoms took up too much room. If I was to make some progress I needed to feel better. So I had to develop and perform techniques to relieve the dyspepsia and the IBS. The well-being I found in these techniques transformed my exercises into shortcuts, not only towards a physical but also towards a social, emotional and psychological well-being.

The shortcuts I describe are what give the book its original character. This is how I hope to be able to help, without falling into the hell of good intentions, without trying to save the world, or experiencing problems with helping relationships. I feel that the distance created by the act of writing allows me communicate my shortcuts and touch readers who may need it in their "private lives."

3 – My Approach

MY PSYCHOANALYSIS

It was through psychoanalysis that I finally managed to unravel my relationship with my own body. Until then I thought that my discomfort had a life of its own like a disease, something mysterious that kept growing until finally it took up so much space that I had to deal with it, or that was detrimental to my quality of life. I realized that I was asking my body to solve a great deal of my problems, including the emotions my mother had taught me to ignore, so that I wouldn't have to suffer. For example, when there was a family visit planned I had to ask myself if I should stand my ground and avoid the reunion or, like a good boy, show up and then let a week pass before I let my body take stock my digestive system was petrified for four days, I went through insomnia, migraine, nausea, fatigue, depression, and finally… recovery. However, since I was in a relationship, my "purely physical" cycle of control and recovery did affect my relation with my spouse.

There also came a time when, in addition to the symptoms, I felt that my body was unable to put up with me any longer. Even life's smallest pleasures held no interest for me. Every effort and additional demand on my body ended in failure and I needed progressively longer periods to recover. It was not easy for me to clear up this relationship, and even less to review it. I had to re-learn that the body is healthy, that it has its own needs, needs that must be met "regularly" with an almost monastic zeal. I had to learn not to give in at the slightest difficulty, that my body has a personality all its own that I must work with. I also understood that, when faced with a difficult situation, being self-assertive caused the same physical symptoms as when I froze. However, I was definitely more satisfied and my body was recovering more rapidly. It was as if "my inner child" was pleased with the fact that I was self-assertive, even though a difficult situation remains a difficult situation... to recover from.

As I began feeling better, I started a dialogue with what I refer to as "my inner child": "What would you like, what would make you feel better, what would allow me to do what I want?", or, "What would be the consequences of this or that action or thought?". The answers were straightforward, even naive, and similar to what we call common sense. It then became possible for me to clinch a deal with that inner child. It is absolutely essential to respect the agreement, to reward "ourselves" and in that way, to regain that friendship with the inner child, although the possibility of a relapse is always there. We need to become indulgent, patient with one another. However, I was the one who had to be reasonable and self-assertive, who had to make sure I made the right choices, I took my wants and desires into account, as well as my needs and emotions. It was the start of a better relationship. If I neglected it the symptoms resurfaced, along with the sadness. Naturally, it was a struggle to avoid reacting against that inner child, avoid re-opening hostilities. However, now, when I make a decision that is good for both of us, even if it is a difficult or unusual one, I feel a deep joy, and even shivers, binds our agreement.

My inner child has become an excellent advisor, who makes no bones about putting me "symptomatically speaking", in my place. My inner child has improved my relationship with my wife by making me see that her complaints often resembled his. For instance, my wife would ask me, "Why did you freeze in that situation?" My inner child could express that same situation as, "Why did you leave me alone again to be scared and having to take care of that problem by myself?" So, by being a better listener and allowing myself more access to my inner child, I was able to react more rapidly and appropriately. My relationship with my wife has greatly improved: nowadays I almost never hurt myself or make a blunder.

Therefore, my symptoms tell me when something is not right with my life, they reveal my erroneous thoughts (cognitive distortion), or how I react to a particular event, or what comes out of my failure to assert myself. This was even more obvious when I found myself freezing, as I did when I was just a small child. My symptoms, especially the accumulated gases, told me that it was enough, that I needed to take care of myself, that I should "break the deadlock" and begin "moving" again.

I was always afraid of my father. He often looked for excuses to take his anger out on us kids. I hated to be caught, to be "ill-taken." I felt that I needed to always be on the alert to avoid being noticed by him... until the day I realized that I had become hyper-vigilant, that it was my turn to see the "black sheep" in others, that I felt drawn to this kind of situation because I found in it an opportunity for a "significant" relationship. I was also drawn to people who spelled danger, I believed that I could domesticate them, that they would help me anticipate the blows and avoid them. My dangerous relationships allowed me to renew the discomfort, to be on familiar grounds: in short, to be in a lousy relationship with someone "doing things for my own good."

So I started focusing on my emotional and physiological responses. Now, every time I feel uncomfortable, become obsessed or feel myself becoming aggressive "apparently without reason", I ask myself, "Is there something wrong? What part of it is mine (the inner reality), and what part of it has to do with others (outer reality)? Could this be a recurrent feeling, a familiar feeling or a response to my inner reality?" Muriel Schiffman's[1] book is very revealing concerning the good that can emerge from such questioning.

---

[1]   Muriel Schiffman. 1967. *Self Therapy: Techniques for Personal Growth*, Self Therapy Press.

The feeling that something is not quite right is an opportunity I must hang onto. When I realize that what happens is actually an outside event or thing affecting me, I get a deep sense of freedom, of gratitude and power. Although oftentimes I cannot change an outside event, I feel free because I know that my response is not the result of some childhood problem I haven't come to terms with, but a normal reaction to such an event. This should facilitate my self-assertiveness or to let it go if I can't change it, as well as my physical recovery.

The same can also be applied to foods. The discovery of gas-producing foods, their management, allows me to take charge of and treat my symptoms more effectively.

Thus, to proceed further in my analysis I had to learn to take care of every physical discomfort I experienced. Every one of them would take months, even years, to relieve. As I became able to understand what this discomfort was hiding, and as I perfected and repeated my gas and nervous tension evacuation exercises, I was able to advance in my psychoanalysis. Focusing on relieving a discomfort for months at a time is a way to make oneself move, to de-stabilize oneself, to become assertive towards ourselves (self-assertive.) Actually, to be assertive towards others means letting them know what we like, demanding a change in behaviour. To be assertive towards ourselves means putting ourselves in a situation where we can become different, where we ask ourselves, even require of ourselves that we act and think differently. Now, assertiveness—as when we assert ourselves before someone—mustn't be the result of a projection or of an attempt to wreak vengeance or punishment. If this is the case, the outcome will not be positive, and we may be tempted to abandon any attempt at assertiveness. It takes time, patience and judgement to determine if self-assertiveness is the result of constructive behaviour. I experienced the same thing when I was treating my symptoms. Often, the result was not immediate. As well, my focus on a specific symptom was likely to increase the discomfort or sensation related to that symptom.

Moreover, there was anxiety to manage. Even if my ability to manage a symptom became associated with increased self-knowledge, the elimination of that symptom invariably led to deeper ones that had been imperceptible until then. I ended up being afraid of totally relieving a symptom because I dreaded the symptom(s) that it would uncover.

Moreover, a gastric disorder caused by a virus, the flu or serious fatigue could cloud the issue. I had to learn to differentiate psycho-somatic discomfort and purely physical discomfort. However, once this issue is clarified it is easier to focus only on what is likely to alleviate a physical symptom, to be more confident when taking a "shortcut."

In this way I was able to tackle the body's symbolism. With patience, the body's language is finally transformed into "I", which eventually occupies more space, incorporates more parameters. For instance, a contraction of the colon systematically occurs when a person says something offensive to me, to put it plainly, makes a "bitchy" comment. I then have to manage everything at once, the physical pain caused by this as well as the psychological and relational aspects. It can be extremely demanding, even colossal work, but in my case the results were highly rewarding. At last, I am no longer the victim of my symptoms. So, when a symptom turns up I systematically ask myself the five following questions: "What did I eat recently?"; "How long has it been since I did my gas and nervous tension evacuation exercises?"; "Am I tired (did I sleep well recently?)"; "Does this remind me of something (an old symptom, for example?)"; "Was I the butt of a bitchy comment or did I meet someone or encounter a difficult situation recently?" Every one of these questions must be examined, and I must find a suitable answer for each. After this is done, all I need to do is apply one of the appropriate remedies.

I wanted to avoid the traditional medical approach as much as possible. I was under the impression that medical doctors, by prescribing medicines had me — and my inner mystery — under their power, and that the time spent with them did not help me understand the cause of my discomfort. I wanted to learn how to know myself and how to treat myself. When I was very young, I felt that doctors were in collusion with my parents, so naturally I was afraid of them: "Treatment can hurt!" I didn't want the doctor to know my abdomen, my foundation, as Dr Devroede would say.

One day, during a session with my psychoanalyst, as I was complaining about my abdominal pain and she suggested that I see a doctor, she told me that the abdomen was intended *"to move."* In other words, that it wasn't normal to have so much abdominal pain. This comment gave me food for thought but better still, it helped me develop a bond of trust with my body. With regard to intestinal pain, it became possible for me to loosen up, to let go — since this is what the abdomen is meant to do — to stop holding it in for fear of experiencing even more pain. It was as if, through her, my mother was telling me that, even if I did let go, nobody would cause me pain anymore.

That is how the importance of taking care of our body was gradually revealed to me. The notion of self-treatment of abdominal pain was taking shape. To parody Dr Peck, who developed the hypothesis of a psychology of evil, I kept on searching and I understood that I could overcome "my" own evil (abdominal pain).

FOR WHOM IS THIS BOOK INTENDED?

Studies have shown that nearly a third of all people suffer from gastric problems at some point in their lives. Such chronic and severe problems can make your life a living hell. The horizon begins to shrink: I can't eat this or that, I can't exercise because I feel terrible either during or after; I can't go to parties, on trips, I can't go out... Eating or drinking too much is forbidden, everything becomes unbearable, etc.

Naturally, this book is intended for people who suffer from gastric reflux, stomach and intestinal gas, slow digestion, hiccups, some types of backache, as well as alternating diarrhoea and constipation, migraines and insomnia. Someone may have gastric problems for years and not even know it. People who are aware that they have this problem can reap benefits of reading this book sooner.

A simple approach, one that is likely to give positive results, can benefit those who suffer from FDDs. I think that, in some cases, people who have malformations or who suffer from an inflammatory disease can also benefit from gas-expelling exercises in the digestive system.

The activity and availability of the nervous system are extremely demanding. Pain reduces availability, which is crucial to creativity, proper care, a rewarding social and work lives, the ability to let go. When things are not working well we turn to our defence mechanisms or to medications. Relaxation techniques may eventually reduce the need for medications and improve our general well-being.

People who suffer from excess nervous tension are likely to develop psychosomatic symptoms, such as migraines. Their presence is a source of stress in itself. These people can turn to relaxation to relieve fatigue and nervous tension, but also to help evacuate gas and treat other symptoms. It is however very difficult to relax when you are suffering from FDDs related symptoms.

If one is to benefit from quality sleep, favourable conditions must be present. The presence of gas, of various symptoms, retention or excess nervous tension affects our sleep. It is possible to find quality sleep by dealing with each of these symptoms. At the same time, insomnia, or the return of insomnia, is a sign that something isn't right. By using the proper treatments we can improve our sleeping conditions considerably.

Through toilet training we are taught all the benefits of adequate retention for life in society. However, when it turns into a preferred lifestyle, a manner of living, thinking and relating to our body, it eventually slows us down, bogs us down: the basic needs are held in, gas can accumulate. We learn how to hold in tensions, headaches, emotions, assertiveness, etc. The nervous system learns how to unload itself in a way that appears to the patient to be unconscious (discomfort, migraine, aggressiveness, fantasy world, tantrums, hysteria.) It is therefore essential to develop an approach to help reduce the automatism of retention or its excesses as much as possible.

What I found extremely satisfying when I developed the gas-expelling technique was that I was able to greatly improve our son's quality of life. It is my belief that he sleeps better than I did at his age, he has more confidence in life and I think he feels that his parents can do something for him. This book is therefore also intended for the parents of children with stomach problems.

Release gas and nervous tension can complete well doctors and therapists' remedies, especially when their interventions fail. It helps relieve symptoms directly and, above all, to sometimes reduce our dependency on medicines and surgery. As an example, I suffered from a disc hernia in 1997. Without the repeat gas-expelling exercises and my relaxation technique I believe I would have had to go under the knife. These methods can also help patients become more self-sufficient.

DIAGNOSIS

This section describes **my own perception** of the symptoms associated with gas accumulation (reflux, dyspepsia and IBS), nervous tension and pain as I experience them. A more technical description of these symptoms is discussed in the section "Review of Literature". Although my experience, and the comments made by several readers, confirm the need to evacuate gas from the stomach and the large intestine, this approach is not recognized by medicine. It therefore represents my personal contribution. Since there is so little scientific coverage of this issue, I devote special attention to it. As for nervous tension and pain, these factors are recognized by medicine as being FDDs components, and there are medical solutions for these complaints. In this case, my personal contribution is to describe the natural techniques I practice to relieve them.

• For gas in the stomach and the large intestine

One of the signs that gas accumulates in the digestive system is heartburn, which can occur when we are intensely occupied or preoccupied, or simply when we have eaten a meal that is not well balanced, or a vegetarian meal when we are not used to it. When I was young, a gulp of soft drink was enough to give me painful heartburn. Feeling bloated or persistently hungry while being unable to eat anything also point to this condition, and so do recurrent indigestion and nausea. For me, the occasional hiccups are the body's attempt to release stomach gas.

The feeling of heaviness, of fullness, of being stuffed that follow a meal, often hides the presence of gas. Irregularity, diarrhoea and constipation, intestinal cramps and colic are also a sign that gas is present.

Cold hands or feet, frequently waking up with a start during the night (dreams) or at the slightest touch or noise, can also be the result of gas accumulation. An empty feeling, stress that nothing can relieve, being intolerant, bouts of anxiety can also be caused by gas accumulation.

Back pain that is not persistent, sciatic pain, cramps in the calves can also indicate gas accumulation. "When the bowel is locked into a cramp, the fecal matter does not move along as it should, yet the water in the fecal matter keeps getting absorbed into the intestinal wall causing constipation. Air can become trapped inside a section of cramping, causing swelling, bloating, and abdominal pain.[2]" On the cardiovascular and respiratory levels, gas can cause momentary arrhythmia, an oppressive feeling, the inability to breathe deeply (thoracic breathing.)

Moreover, the accumulation of gas has often produces dizziness, tinnitus, even spasms and tics. It can generate silent gastric reflux

---

[2]   Carolyn Dean, M.D., ND and L. Christine Wheeler, MA. IBS for Dummies. Wiley Publishing, Inc., Hobeken NJ, 2006. p. 53.

which can lead to an irritation of the respiratory tract, including laryngitis and pharyngitis.

Finally, on the psychological level, hysteria, paranoid tendencies (I don't feel well, somebody is against me), irritability, a desire to be still (not making waves), wishing to avoid any form of exercise, can also be exacerbated by the presence of gas.

- **For excess nervous tension**

Several of the symptoms I mentioned earlier can be related to a build-up of nervous tension. In my case, excess nervous tension ended up affecting my musculature. I was growing weaker and often sprained my wrists, my ankles or my back. Massages, including antigymnastics and physical therapy, help relax the muscles, reduce some of the tension, but it is not enough to eliminate the tension message circulated by the nervous system.

In general, we hear that excess nervous tension has psychological, social or economic causes. Experience has taught me that discomfort, excess bloating for example, leads to a feeling of urgency, as if the body anticipated imminent danger. The nervous system apparently reacts as if there was no solution possible. Then, since the symptoms won't go away, an underlying feeling of panic develops. Here again, a simple solution must be found to reduce the tension at its source, if possible: in this case, the solution would be to treat the bloating.

Insomnia is a sign of excess tension but it can also be caused by the presence of accumulated gas. Finally, in my case, excess nervous tension manifests itself by impatience, which can sometimes become dangerous especially for me or by a lack of psychological availability. It is also the cause of many distractions and revealing blunders.

MY HYPOTHESES

In this chapter I take stock of hypotheses that, I believe, can explain the presence of FDDs. Like Gilles Vigneault in his song "Paulu Gazette", "When we know the names of things... we possess them!" Many people who suffer from FDDs are searching, often with the help of health care professionals, for the cause of their discomfort. In the "Review of Literature" section, I list some of these hypotheses and the approaches that may be used to treat these discomforts. Unfortunately, I learned through personal experience that merely knowing the cause of a discomfort doesn't relieve it. However, it can help reassure and, above all, provide the appropriate care.

- **For the gas**

Although we have the benefit of a varied diet all year round, our food habits, especially with regard to the so convenient processed foods, can be hard to digest. Potato chips, gluten-based foods (bread, cakes, bagels, pastry, etc.), as well as soft drinks, impress me as being gas-generating foods. It should be pointed out that legumes and some vegetables such as cauliflower, corn and broccoli are known to generate gas. Sugar can be a source of fermentation.

Therefore, we must learn to be aware of our inability to tolerate particular foods. However, I believe that the fact that our system cannot tolerate a wide variety of foods indicates a problem with gas. But it is not that easy to identify a food intolerance problem. There is a chapter in the "Review of Literature" that distinguishes between the notions of allergy and food intolerance. One of the clues to identifying a food allergy as the culprit for diarrhoea is the presence of other histamine hitchhikers like hives, asthma, eczema, and nasal discharge[3]. Moreover, studies show that some people swallow air as they eat, which can easily be remedied. If such is the case, we could be tempted to wrongly attribute our gas problems with foods we have

---

[3]   Ibid, p. 69.

recently eaten. On average, less than one fifth of IBS patient who think they have food intolerance are confirmed by studies.

There is a wide range of literature, of uneven quality, about the benefits of healthy eating. Food issues will not be discussed extensively in this book. Doctors often refer their patients to dieticians. The damaging effects of eating gas-generating food, as well as food our body doesn't tolerate, may be offset effectively by eating less of them. However, I do believe that we can eat these foods in moderation if we perform the gas-expelling exercises. My experience has shown me that, once gas has been eliminated from the digestive system I can handle a wide variety of foods, even those that are gas-generating. On the other hand, it also seems to me that gases are just the result of normal digestive process. So they can accumulate in the digestive track even though we try to avoid all foods that could trigger them.

The "gas" issue can be traced back to our early childhood. Many parents have been taught that infants need to be burped. It doesn't take much negligence for a child to suffer from colic. If the situation persists, the child's body adapts to it. Even though as the child ages he or she becomes stronger and gets some sleep, the nights can be restless, with frequent waking periods. As regards toilet training, when care is delayed or painful, to the child it can mean that relief will be a source of problem. He can get into the habit—as I did—of holding everything in as long as possible, and may never feel really well. This also occurs when children, out of boredom, entertain themselves by holding it in and "playing with their insides." It is mentioned in literature that the simple fact of holding it in can cause constipation lasting up to a week.

Bacterial flora often contains *helicobacter pylori*, which is transmitted through the saliva and can cause stomach ulcers. Antibiotics have the potential to eradicate it. It is important to see a doctor, who will detect the condition easily by a simple drugstore test. On a trip it is possible to get food poisoning. These problems are discussed later.

The problems caused by a sedentary lifestyle cannot be overestimated. This lifestyle is largely involved in what I call the "accumulation phase." The less we move, the more gas accumulates. Diffuse discomfort increases, becomes more complicated to the point where moving becomes painful. To want to start moving again can even be agonizing.

I was able to experiment that a change in internal acidity level can create gas problems. However, this hypothesis is not medically recognized. Too much alkalinity (which can be caused by a diet rich in vegetables and pasta) is conducive to infections, colic and diarrhoea. One can easily detect an acidobasic problem by using the short sticks available in hospitals and health food stores, or simply by the smell and the opacity of urine. Many times a simple diet adjustment will suffice. On the other hand, an alkalinity problem can also be caused by a large accumulation of gas, which leads to diarrhoea and kidney dysfunction.

Paradoxically, in my case, when my system is alkaline, the resulting accumulation of stomach gas stretches the walls of the stomach, causing heartburn. Taking an antacid to relieve the condition can be especially counterproductive since it increases my system's alkalinity. Therefore, taking antacids ultimately creates a vicious circle. In parallel, too much acidity irritates the digestive system and can also cause heartburn. To compensate for it we have to eat food that is alkaline. When there is heartburn a good diagnosis is crucial in determining the proper treatment.

Regarding pre-menstrual or preovulatory symptoms, my wife has noticed that during this period she regularly has digestive problems, is more sensitive to particular foods and has more gas.

Finally, I should mention a predisposition towards the psychosomatic reactions of the digestive system. Stress is known to noticeably slow down the stomach's movements (motility.) For many people, unpleasant events or relationships are dealt with on the inside. Such slowing down of the digestive system is conducive to gas accumulation.

• For nervous tension

I tend to believe that people who suffer from excess gas have primarily a problem with the build-up of nervous tension. That doesn't mean that all people suffering from stress will develop IBS. The digestive system is designed to function normally. Excepting the presence of abnormalities, tension can cause our digestive system to work in slow motion, causing diarrhoea and constipation in alternation. Thus, excess gas suggests a tendency to accumulate nervous tension.

People who are already taking medication to relieve pain or to slow down, those who have high blood pressure or who suffer from psychosomatic diseases or migraines are at a high risk of accumulating nervous tension.

Other symptoms are indicators of excess tension. Wanting to be left alone (not wanting to be around other people), pain in the eyes, neck, shoulders, back ... can be related to excessive tension. Feeling that our digestive system is upside down, slow or stagnant is also a sign of excess tension. To be constantly thinking without any results, to be regularly obsessed, unsure of your own judgment, also signal excess tension. To feel that life is passing you by, that you are beside yourselves, not able to listen to your body; to have persistent pain and muscular tension, tics and manias; or when good intentions too often yield negative results are also signs. Feeling bubbled up[4], outside of your own skin, is another sign. As well as being unable to let go although we know that it may be the best solution.

---

[4] When I am full of gas, I tell myself that "I am busy", in the sense that the phone is busy, and that I am out of touch with myself. I feel that I am cut off from my body: I become shut in mentally, far from my heart. My wife and I have a code: "Go and get some rest, dear, you're all bubbled up!" It's hard on my pride, but everything returns to normal once I've done my exercises. We don't cut off communication, we merely postpone it. It is a good way for us to avoid misunderstandings and conflicts.

• **Visceral hypersensitivity**

Accumulated gas and excess nervous tension do not lead to gastrointestinal discomfort for everyone. Visceral hypersensitivity is one of the diagnostic criteria. Scientific tests have shown that people who suffer from FDDs, like migraine sufferers, have a heightened perception of discomfort or pain with the same stimuli, whether this involves the intestines or the skin. However, it is increasingly recognized that people who complain about FDDs are not any more "whiny" than others.

Logically, releasing gas and nervous tension should heighten the feeling of well-being in people who suffer from FDDs. My experience tells me that visceral hypersensitivity is what takes longer to improve, especially without medications. However, regularly performing the exercises I suggest builds up a feeling of self-confidence and ease over the long run. This is because my techniques are constantly becoming more effective, or could it be that a slow decrease in my visceral sensitivity comes into play? I'm not sure. What I can say is that, as time goes by, I get the impression that I feel increasingly better and that I am more and more able "to take it!"

RESISTANCE

• **The "forbidden" eructation and flatulence**

Putting it mildly, in Western societies eructation and farting are considered rude and unacceptable: children are taught early that they should not do these things, especially in public. Yet, those needs are as essential as urinating and defecating, which we also have to hold in, but which can be relieved in a manner and at a time that is considered appropriate, plus, they are not as shameful.

Some highly disgraceful epithets can be attached to one who belches and farts. Therefore, many who have gas try to hold onto it. Even worse, the "suppression" gets to be a habit such that we end up feeling we don't have gas at all. In such a context a person can even become ill, steadily weaker and finally weigh heavily on relatives and society. The book entitled *Éloge du pet* ("In praise of farts"), by Mercier de Compiègne, deals humorously with this aspect.

So then, toilet training and decorum compel people to hide, delay relief, ignore their body and neglect themselves. We live in a closed-up, motionless world with a pessimistic view of ourselves and of the future. The depressive potential of severe FDDs symptoms should not be underestimated. A person suffering from excess gas often has to be patient and keep hoping that the healing will come by itself... as we used to do with the small hurts of our early childhood. This person may seek treatment for secondary symptoms and remain anxious for a long time, not knowing what is "happening inside."

• For nervous tension

Talking about our inner tensions, about anguish, anxiety and stress can be a bigger taboo than talking about the venereal diseases resulting from our sexual prowess. It is considered a sign of weakness. For society at large, for co-workers or for the family it is the individual who is at fault, who would feel better if only he or she would make the necessary efforts, that is, think and act like the rest of us.

There is also the trend towards globalization, which creates an ever-increasing urgency to adjust, adapt, and perform. Those who cannot adapt have to make way for the others! It is as if there should be a purgatory, a limbo from which people would emerge once they were ready to join in the parade. In a way, I feel that we are living in a period where the *pecking order* prevails, where the slightest weakness is reason enough to kick us out. Poor souls of the new world order be discreet!

• Rejecting the values and practices of the past

Nowadays, some behaviours of traditional societies are viewed as helpful in promoting good health. First, we should mention physical activity. In former times, there were very few of the things that facilitate modern life (kitchen appliances, farm equipment, automobiles, etc.) For many people, walking has even become a pastime, a luxury, because you have to spend time doing it. When people lived out of doors more it was easier for them to relieve themselves, especially when they needed to belch or fart. In the Middle Ages, sacred holidays allowed people almost as much "free time" as we have today. Religious activities helped foster social integration and harmony, as well as the feeling of well-being that came with the Sacrament of Penance. Prayers allowed people to let go and confront their problems from a spiritual rather than a personal perspective. People also refer to the loss of the sense of celebration, of folkloric dances, etc.

• **Our resistances (What purpose do they serve?)**

Our discomforts are so much a part of ourselves, they are so well integrated in our personality that, sometimes, seeing them disappear is like being thrown into the unknown. We may ask ourselves what our character would be like if we were feeling better.

We draw some benefits from our discomforts. We can use our discomforts to attract attention, as an assertiveness tool, to refuse to pay attention to others or even to dispel boredom. The absence of discomforts forces us to be happy, to work, to have a social life, to be compassionate.

When we have gas with hypersensitivity we are confined to a personalized, limited vision of things, being unavailable to the outside world. It is as if we developed an "intestinal", a short-sighted vision. On a psychological level it means being isolated, without compromise. A being to whom we can't ask anything, someone who is "pre-occupied"... with his or her digestion. Having too much gas also means feeling full. We may get the impression that we experience a kind of peace, an absence of struggle for survival (fullness), a rest from the tension created by hunger.

Having gas means being tense, it also means constantly having to cope on our own instead of being assertive towards the outside, others and ourselves, it is our unconscious, our body that has to cope. The body, helpless, is distressed because of the struggles, and most of all, because of the intestinal pain that it must cope with. Being non-assertive means being doomed to feeling unwell. Our unconscious is then forced to manipulate us to get some satisfaction. So we become victims of ourselves, locked in a vicious circle.

Another reason for not doing anything is the demand and sometimes the pain that we have to assume with self-treatment. As Dr Oppenheim would say, it is so much simpler to take a pill. Taking care of ourselves, especially being persistent, is a demanding task. If, as the saying goes, there is no beauty without pain, the same also applies to improving our condition.

The book IBS for Dummies[5] refers to a 2004 study by Italian doctors that shows that people with IBS are not able to expel intestinal gas. For them, it seems that people with IBS have a special attachment to gas and don't like to let it go. With a large amount of gas stuck in your system, it is normal to feel uncomfortable. That causes bowel to stretch, creating abdominal pain. For these doctors, pressure stretching the rectal area activates some areas of the brain, which makes people feel more symptoms. In my view, we then have at least to learn to let it go!

Emerging from our discomforts, accepting and going beyond our resistances and those of society to treat ourselves is truly a feat. Sometimes, an illness or a failure may force us to take better care of ourselves. In his book, *Les tremblements intérieurs* (p. 23), Dr Daniel Dufour recalls the words of Laura, one of his patients, who tells him, "Without this disease I would not be feeling as well as I am feeling today, both morally and physically!" Treating ourselves, when we tend to somatise, can make us go through very painful, even agonizing periods, without even knowing what the outcome will be.

---

[5]   Ibid, p. 24.

Like I would often say while I followed therapy, we know what we leave, but we don't know what we will get from it.

For those who are indisposed because of gas, nervous tension and the pain associated with FDDs, I hope that the exercises that follow will improve your quality of life. Some readers have told me that my testimonial, and the mere fact of knowing that, "it is now permitted to release ourselves" did them a lot of good. I want to introduce you to the art of "releasing" yourself, of setting yourself free!

EXPELLING GAS FROM THE STOMACH

• A few assumptions

When you don't feel well, when you feel pain in your abdomen, in your body, is there a simple, mechanical approach that can be developed or suggested to alleviate this pain? In fact, gas release is based on fairly simple assumptions:

- Gas tends to rise in a liquid environment;
- The content of the stomach and large intestine is carried from the mouth to the rectum (therefore, in an opposite direction from the direction of the gas in a liquid environment; I refer here to the stomach and right section of the large intestine);
- Gas can get trapped and accumulate in the digestive tract (up to four litres of air in the stomach), restricting the flow of gas, obstructing the intestines and causing a high level of discomfort that can be long-lasting, even cramps;
- Nervous tension hinders the flow of gas (through contraction), but gas itself provoke a sense of pain or inner danger with triggers nervous tension;
- If the air volume in the digestive system is significant, unjamming the gas or, better yet, expelling it improves motility and greatly reduces discomfort (in my case, I

simply manage to eliminate as much as possible, which means a lot).

• Belching

Belching is natural, yet some people - I used to be one of them - cannot manage it. When a person is unable to belch, the gas has to be expelled through the intestines, which means that it builds up and forms pockets along the digestive tract. Fortunately, you can learn to belch on demand, i.e., force yourself to belch in a number of ways. The easiest and better known method is the belching contests teenagers engage in. **What you need to do is focus, relax your throat and abdomen and take a deep breath as you inflate your abdomen as much as possible while holding the air inside your lungs and inflated abdomen, then swallow a small air bubble and then push it out immediately through the mouth.** Ideally, more air should come out through the mouth than what was swallowed at first. These are the basics of the gas release technique. After it becomes a habit it is enough to just swallow a small air bubble and expel it.

There is a variation to this technique, which makes it even more effective: you contract your pectoral muscles after swallowing an air bubble. This increases the internal pressure of the stomach and forces out the air that has built up. The pressure variation (contracting-releasing) also promotes the flow of gas in the large intestine.

This belching mechanism works because, when we try to force out the small air bubble that has just been swallowed, some of the air contained in the stomach is added to this air bubble. I perfected my technique over the years to the point where I could swallow as little air as possible to generate a belch, and make the most of the air expelled along with the air bubble.

Here is another way to generate big belches. After lying in a hot bath for a few minutes I relax my abdomen and inflate it as gently as possible while taking a deep breath. I then breathe out while loosening up my abdomen. I do this breathing exercise four or five times. Then, after breathing deeply while inflating and loosening the abdomen, I slowly pull myself up to a sitting position. Generally, this causes the air to rise considerably. If it doesn't rise of its own accord, I swallow a small air bubble. Usually, this is enough. You can also do it sitting on the couch or rocking back and forth. This technique can be repeated a many times.

A very effective way to expel gas is by hiccupping. From my experience, a hiccup is a strong contraction of the diaphragm caused by the body's attempt to release excess gas trapped in the pit of the stomach. However, these movements are random. You can learn to direct the gas displaced by hiccups towards the upper part of the stomach. This causes a large amount of gas to rise rapidly. However, when the gas moves upward it can be painful. With practice, you will manage to do it with very little pain.

Since hiccups are caused by too much gas, hiccupping to expel the gas will eliminate the cause. When I release gas that the hiccups have caused to rise, the hiccups only last for a short time. With practice I managed to make the hiccups last longer (I maintain diaphragm contractions) by inflating the abdomen to expel as much gas as I possibly can. I consider that two to three minutes of belching, with the hiccups, gets the same results as up to twenty minutes of the gas release exercises.

On the other hand, if you already have a problem with hiccups, you only need to expel the air to make them quickly go away. I feel that my stomach is deeply relaxed at the end of a hiccupping and belching session.

Another effective way of releasing stomach gas is through nausea and throwing up. People suffering from anorexia or bulimia, and even artists who get stage fright, often use this method, voluntarily or not. A general well-being ensues; but this is a fairly radical and painful method and, I should add, not very pleasant. Do we really need to suffer that much to feel better?

Swallowing air when there is already too much of it in the stomach is not a lot of fun, especially if we don't succeed in forcing it out at the beginning. You need to keep trying. You can also drink a glass of water or two; the water dilutes the stomach bowl so air passes through it more easily. Don't forget that dehydratation provokes gas production in the digestive track.

Another way is to loosen up your upper abdomen as much as you can by taking a few deep breaths. Belching requires a specific posture, a specific orientation of the upper body. Leaning forward slightly or stretching your neck can also help. If you can't manage it, either your spouse, one of your older children or an acquaintance, who may be good at this, can give you a demonstration! Learning to take care of you is well worth a laugh!

Generally, at first, swallowing an air bubble only yields small belches. When the upper part of the stomach is relaxed and you have refined your technique, the ascent of the gas (rumbling noises) will be that more significant. Hearing a rumbling noise after belching is a sign that the technique is working. With practice, I hear this noise almost every time I belch. On the other hand, even with good control, the rising of the gas varies greatly. I tell myself that there are no bad belches: even when I pass only a small quantity of air, I better myself.

Repeated belching reduces the pressure in the upper part of the stomach. The deeply trapped gas tends to rise to restore the inner balance. I call "fluid mechanics" the upward movement of air wedged at the bottom of the stomach against the flow of the food; it is quicker when the pressure at the top of the stomach is lower than at the bottom.

Experience has shown me that it is relatively easy to release the air pockets that have accumulated in the upper and middle parts of the stomach, using belching, naturally. The air pockets lodged in the lower part of the stomach are unfortunately much more difficult to force out. However, I feel that, when released they yield the highest benefits. In fact, the air pockets resting in the pit of the stomach tend to obstruct the lower part of the large intestine and paralyse gas movements. Once this air is released, the large intestine lets out numerous rumbling noises. We will get back to this further on.

To locate the area where the gas is lodged in the stomach, I take a deep breath. I focus to feel where the most painful place is located in the abdomen. This will point out the area where the gas is possibly trapped. Another way to localise the gas is to listen to the rumbling noises. Generally, they make themselves heard precisely where the air has just been released, which often coincides with the area where the most intense pain is felt. I belch systematically after every rumbling noise emitted by the stomach: it would be useless to belch after a rumbling noise emitted by the large intestine. Once the air is released, I take a deep breath again and, most of the time, I no longer feel or feel less pain where the rumbling first started.

I then look for another painful area. I try to relax the abdomen as much as I can to facilitate the unjamming of the air lodged in that area. Often, especially at the bottom of the stomach, the air is not released immediately. Sometimes, it takes from two to three deep breaths and as many relaxation movements before I can feel release. Generally, when I take a deep breath, I hold the ballooning of the belly as much as I can do leaving room for gas movements. While I expire, I wait and I try to relax for as long as I can near the area identified as the most painful. If the gas hasn't been loosened up, I inspire, take a few regular breaths and then again take a deep breath and so on between ballooning and relaxing. I keep this up until the gas is released. I hunt down gases wherever I can feel the pain, sometimes for hours.

Another thing we have to learn is how to differentiate between rumbling noises from the stomach and those from the large intestine. In general, the rumbling gets started in the large intestine, on the right side of the abdomen, and then moves left and up, while on the left side of the abdomen the rumbling travels from top to bottom. Contrary to what happens in the case of the stomach, a strong rumbling noise from the large intestine does not cause a significant emission of gas during a forward belch. A stomach rumbling always goes from bottom up, so ending near the oesophagus where it will be easy to expel with the belching technique. These are ways to tell them apart.

When the gas is first released, there may be a slight discomfort. Since the abdomen must be relaxed, I may even feel more discomfort (hypersensitivity). The remedy may seem at first glance worse than the pain itself. Don't worry; the benefits of a total release are well worth this slight momentary discomfort. I just mention it to encourage you to trying again and persevere, if that momentary discomfort appears to be in your first trials of belching technique.

As I begin to practice, and during periods of great crises (anxiety, indigestion, colic, insomnia, gastritis, etc.), I may have to belch for more than two hours to fully loosen up. Later, however, my stomach, intestines, kidneys and blood flow all function smoothly and painlessly. I also recover quality sleep, without restlessness.

Getting rid of the gas in the stomach takes time because it has to be expelled in a direction opposite to the way the digestive system usually push them. If only the upper part of the stomach is released, air will still remain in the depths of the stomach. If this occurs the only relief we get is from heartburn, which isn't bad, come to think of it. To get the maximum effect from this exercise you must expel as much gas as possible to untangle the entire digestive track.

As well, you may suffer from abdominal pain without having a problem with stomach gases. Here again, one way to check if you have stomach gases is to swallow an air bubble. If the bubble takes a while to go down to the stomach, and you can hear it go down along your oesophagus with a relatively constant, high-pitch sound, you may not have a gas problem. In my case, it doesn't take long before the bubble reaches the stomach, and the gas comes up quickly and over a short distance.

• Belching while lying down

Little or no time to take care of myself, a poor diet, a recent stress, meeting people who make me feel bad, all those things can trigger discomfort in the middle of the night (insomnia, anxiety, a tingling sensation, waking up with a start, palpitations, tinnitus ringing in the ears, etc.). When this happens I invariably get up, go and have a pee and drink some liquid, preferably water. Back in bed, I sit and belch for a few minutes to release the upper part of the stomach. Then, I lay down, alternating my right and left sides, sometimes with a rocking movement, and I belch in that position. While resting on the right side of my body I pull my arm up alongside my head and I lift my head with my hand. Then I start belching again in that position. Amazingly, the rumblings – so the air – then will come from the right side of the stomach up to the oesophagus.

Sometimes if I also feel muscle tension in the legs, I gently push my head forward. I also fold my right leg and place my left heel under my right knee. Using my left hand, I grab my right ankle and pull it towards my backside (guaranteed stretching). The right side of my back is generally tenser than my left. I take advantage of this to stretch my entire right side while belching.

After three to five minutes on one side, I straighten up and belch several times. When I sit down to belch, it often happens that a lot of gas rises up (big rumbling noises). Then, I lie down on the opposite side. In this case let's say the left. I still pull my arm up alongside my head and I lift again my head with my hand and I start belching. As you can predict, the rumbling and gas will part from the left side of my stomach upward. After three to five minutes of belching, I sit and belch again. Normally, an hour of this alternate treatment is well enough to release air of my stomach entirely. Generally I don't spend as much time belching when lying on my right side. I occasionally alternate between the sitting position and lying on my left side a few times.

The loosening up of gas from the upper stomach, while lying on my right side, is very useful because it helps reduce the pressure on the large intestine. Releasing gas from the large intestine becomes easier as a result.

I repeat this exercise four to eight times according to the quantity of gas I feel is trapped, or until I feel sufficiently relaxed to be sure I can fall asleep. In fact, with experience and trial and error, I know when I will be able to fall into a deep sleep. If I haven't released enough gas I simply cannot go back to sleep. Generally, it is when the gas at the bottom of the stomach, especially on the left side, is released that I manage to fall asleep.

Sometimes I interrupt the cycle by resting on my stomach for a short while. This allows me to release gas from the large intestine more easily. Some time may elapse before I feel the need to expel gas.

I can also belch lying down on my back, but it took me several years to manage it. Generally, I belch after having released the gas from the stomach almost completely. I let out a few belches, and usually fall into a deep sleep.

Belching in every one of these positions helps expel the air lodged in a specific area of the stomach. The sitting position helps release the front of the stomach and the gas trapped at the bottom of the stomach. On my back, I release gases that are close to the back, in the upper part of the stomach. This helps eliminate some of the back pain caused by the gas that may be lodged near the diaphragm. With experience you will feel where exactly in the stomach the gases are trapped. For example, if I feel that there is still gas left deep on the left side of the stomach, I make more belching while lying on that side.

Generally, the more sleep I get before doing my exercises the easiest they will be, and the less time I will require to do them before I go back to sleep. When I am in the middle of a crisis, however, I can wake up after only an hour after going to bed. It takes me a lot longer to expel the air from my digestive system and especially to get it to loosen up. The extent and quality of my sleep before I wake up is an indication of the quantity of air trapped. If I wake up after an hour of sleep I will require at least two hours of exercises to expel the air. Waking up after four hours of sleep requires barely thirty minutes of exercises before I can fall once again into a deep sleep. However, the more gases I manage to expel during the day, the less I will need to do it during the night, and therefore the more sleep I will enjoy before waking up.

In very rare occasions I sleep through the night without waking up. Often, it is the need to urinate that will wake me up. I immediately go and relieve myself. It's no use trying to go back to sleep when this occurs because I will then sleep restlessly. Generally, I find that belching for twenty minutes or so enables me to go back to sleep. Sometimes I wake up with a start or, even worse, with ringing in my ears. In that case, I have to do my exercises for at least two hours to get the symptoms gone. In addition to belching, stretching and respiratory exercises, I also apply my nervous tension release exercises (see below). This shows that treating dyspepsia is possible but demanding. Belching is thorough work which brings invaluable results that I can no longer do without.

• We need a place and time just to ourselves

Ideally, belching is something we can do by ourselves, whether in the car, when walking, watching television or rocking back and forth. I also manage to do it in public transport. In fact, buses or train make so much noise that I can belch discretely without anyone noticing. Most often, however, I belch in the middle of the night.

Naturally, belching for two hours in the middle of the night means that you need to have your own room. For people who live as a couple, it may seem difficult to contemplate this possibility. You will probably have to assert yourself, put across the view that you don't feel well, that this is not the other person's fault, and that it doesn't mean you want a separation. With a room of your own it is easier to relax sufficiently to get a good idea of how you feel and, of course, do the exercises.

I changed job in 2010 and I suffered stress and I had more adaptation difficulties that I thought. To help me I became more zealous about practicing my techniques. I practice more before going to bed for a better sleep night. I go 30 to 45 minutes alone outside on my balcony for belching and relaxing on a rocking chair. I have then a better sleep night. I found also that I had much more gas left in my GI track in the morning that I was expecting to. Hopefully burping is easy in the morning while the stomach is empty and I am relaxed. Burping then helped me a lot to feel better all day and to adapt to my new situation. I did change my routine for the better. Instead of waiting to be waked up by symptoms in the middle of the night, I just do prepare myself much better to have a good sleep night and feel well all day long.

• **Becoming aware of signs of improvement**

A first sign of improvement in gas release exercises is a relief from the pain (if any) in the oesophagus, although it can start again with the rising of the gases. Another sign that there is improvement is the appearance of the rumbling noises that start from an increasingly deeper area. Another clue is the disappearance of the twinge of pain in my back that may have been caused by gas. A frequent need to urinate after a few minutes suggests an improvement, since the body is no longer accumulating and is letting go. A series of farts occurring within a few minutes means that the stomach gas is no longer pressing or blocking the large intestine. The disappearance of the above-mentioned symptoms, one at a time, is a sign of improvement. As I often say: « Gas expelled no longer hurts! »

It is important to be aware of the level of improvement resulting from breaking wind for sustained, extended periods because it is an immediate reward for our efforts. It encourages perseverance.

The following chart lists the exercises that promote gas release. Some of them can be combined. But first, you need to learn how to belch and relax your abdomen as much as possible. In fact, it is almost impossible to belch and release the gas from deep down if you don't know how to relax your abdomen (see release of nervous tension and relaxation techniques described below). Relaxing your abdomen will help make the flow of gas more fluid and, above all, less painful.

Expelling gases from the bottom of the stomach helps reduce the pressure on the large intestine near the rectum. The flow of intestinal gases and their release will then be easier. To help expel gas from the large intestine you can increase the pressure inside the abdomen by pushing for a few seconds as if you needed to defecate. If there is gas in the rectum, the need to let out a fart will quickly follow.

It works in similar fashion as for the stomach, but in the opposite direction, the pressure change in the bottom of the large intestine allowing gases present in the top part of the large intestine to head for the rectum to restore balance. Once the stomach is free of air and relaxed, I only need five to ten minutes to expel the air from the large intestine. Naturally, when I expel gas from the stomach – which can take up to three hours –, the need to fart can sometimes be felt. Since the gases in the large intestine are generally more painful, I never miss an opportunity to get rid of them. I then start to belch.

When I start to belch I generally don't feel the presence of the gas that has accumulated in the large intestine. It is often after I've belched for about twenty minutes that I begin to feel it. It is as if since the stomach no longer being so bloated it causes the large intestine to inflate gently and become more sensitive. I notice that the gas accumulated in the upper left part of the stomach tends to trap the bend of the large intestine in the upper left of the abdomen. I recommend belching while lying on your left side to help bring down the pressure in this section of the stomach. Since we are talking about the gas located in the top part of the stomach, this gas is among the first to be expelled. I then feel cramps or rumblings in that part of the large intestine. However, the gas often remains trapped until the gas from the rectum and lower colon has been expelled. I can then expel them at the same time as the gas from the bottom of the stomach. After this is done, however, the gas located higher in the large intestine is quickly released.

To release the gas located in the large intestine, you first need to check whether there is gas trapped in the rectum. You can verify by pushing for a few moments as if you try to defecate. Once this gas, if any, is released, the way is then clear for the gas accumulated in the higher part of the large intestine to start circulating. You need only to draw a deep breath and relax the left side of your lower abdomen to feel that the gas trapped in that area is moving towards the exit.

Pushing as if you needed to defecate also facilitates the flow of gas in the large intestine. After pushing, however, you can feel some discomfort since the gas-related symptoms are exacerbated by the movement. However, this helps assess several characteristics of my overall condition. For example, if I am suffering from migraine, to push even for a few seconds will increase the pain. I can assess the degree of somatisation, the improvements resulting from the latest treatments, or whether or not I can tolerate more of it. In the same way, I can assess the extent of the exercises remaining to be done to achieve the desired level of well-being. Pushing can also act as a counterbalance to excessive retention. However, pushing should not be overly done to avoid the risk of haemorrhoids, cramps, or the upward movement of gases in the intestine.

When the air finally begins to flow in the large intestine, you will feel some cramps. The natural tendency is to try and hold on to the pain to avoid being overcome by it. It took me a long time before I was able to understand that it was better to let it go. That's why previously testing my pain threshold by pushing can be helpful. The pain threshold that I can tolerate determines the rapidity of the release. The more I let the pain of the cramp go without tensing up, the easier the air that causes the cramp will move towards the rectum, and the shorter the pain will last.

If I become tense, the air will tend to rise in the large intestine. It will not be expelled, and it may be a long time before it comes back. To avoid holding on to the pain, I focus on the painful area, relax it and visualize the passage of the air towards the rectum. I am always surprised by the effectiveness of this approach.

I sometimes apply pressure on a cramp for some thirty seconds or, ideally, a few centimetres higher, near the ribcage. I place my left thumb on my back and rest my four fingers on the area where I feel the cramp is located. Of course, this is very painful at first but the gases rapidly slide towards the exit. Relaxing the anal area can also keep the air from rising up. With practice, and over time, it becomes less necessary to use pressure. Since I found the means to push down the air of a cramp, I feel that my large intestine is working more freely, and I don't worry about it as much.

Intestinal gas, like anxiety, can be relieved temporarily by lying down on the stomach. The pressure resulting from this position facilitates the flow of blood. As for anxiety, this posture can bring temporary relief and have a reassuring effect. However, it can also generate postural problems, especially in the neck area. This is why I only lie on my stomach for a few minutes, only the time it takes to reassure myself if needed, or to expel a few intestinal gases.

Although I generally perform my exercises during the night, one of the best ways to expel flatulence is physical exercise, especially the frequent bending down and getting up. For example, moving boxes, piling wood, picking up leaves, gardening… are all exercises that produce very "liberating" effects. According to my family physician, a simple way to expel gases from the large intestine is to raise your knees for a few minutes, especially the left one, while sitting or lying down.

Alternating deep breathing with panting also produces good results. As mentioned in the section concerning the stomach, you can also practice deep breathing. Often, deep respiratory movements are sufficient. After a very short time you will feel the intestinal gases rising, and feel the need to expel them. This technique is also very efficient. Later in the book you will come across a chapter on deep breathing. Some experts suggest that this method should be used several times a day. It is always worthwhile to resort to it, since the gases expelled during the day will not disturb your night time sleep.

You should always avoid holding on to gas. This tip alone is worth the price of the book. If you are in a social gathering you can simply step aside to a place where you can release yourself without being noticed. Unfortunately, it is so much easier to hang onto it, avoid stepping out to that isolated place, so much easier to "behave nicely." However, as Mercier de Compiègne tells us in his *Éloge du pet ("In praise of the fart"),* "If someone has the guilty fancy to compress it, smother it and stop it in its progress when it wants to come out, it is so eager to enjoy its full rights, so zealous in defence of freedom, that it can torture the fool-hardy and, in its wrath, even cause him to die."[6]

An American study has shown that holding gas in can result in constipation lasting up to a week. As Mercier de Compiègne would say, "The fart is the father of cheerfulness and equality. It can abolish distances that pride has created between master and servant. It makes the former more affable and gives wit to the latter [...] which leads me to conclude that the fart is the father of joy, health, spirit and freedom. All that remains for me to do is to wish that a society of "farters" may be promptly established [...]. That's all. Farewell."[7]

When I was younger I never suspected how much harm I was doing to myself by keeping everything in. And I did it very often. I had to spend countless efforts and attention to get rid of this bad habit. The instructions are plain: never hold it in!

A fart from beans is gentler that one from stress!

---

[6]   This is an unofficial translation.
[7]   This is an unofficial translation.

Table I		
Exercise to release the gas trapped in the stomach and large intestine		
Exercise	**Description**	**Remark**
1. Breathe as if panting	Take deep breaths (like a woman in labour) while abdomen remains inflated.	The purpose of this exercise is to release the gas thoroughly, and should be done after the gas that sits higher in the stomach has been released.
2. Tap the abdomen	Knead the abdomen quite a bit with your hand (wave-like). Occasionally, tap directly on the areas that still feel tight.	To loosen up the last places that are still tight and difficult to release.
3. Massage the abdomen	Massage the abdomen in a clockwise direction.	Massaging should be thorough while applying considerable pressure.
4. Push	Push (as if you needed to defecate) while bearing down for three to five seconds.	Bearing down increases the pressure in the lower abdomen. Do not push too hard.
5. Perform the "Technique Nadeau" (known primarily in Quebec)	Perform various movements to promote gas circulation. In addition, you can also rock the pelvis forward, backward and sideways.	Ten minutes of belching every day while performing the "Technique Nadeau" helps release the higher part of the stomach. It compensates for inactivity.
6. Rock back and forth (highly recommended)	Use a rocking chair while relaxing the abdomen. You can also rock back and forth sitting on a straight back chair.	This simple, comfortable activity stimulates digestion and gas movements.

7. Take advantage of solitary moments	While driving, waiting for the bus, walking, jogging, all are good opportunities to silently belch.	For example, driving and belching for twenty minutes or so prevents heartburn and prolongs sleep. It is also a good way to get ready for a stressful meeting.
8. Laugh or practise laughter therapy	Laughing causes spasmodic contractions throughout the body. Some people belch inadvertently when they laugh.	You can tickle a child (not too much) who has trouble falling asleep. Laughter therapy is a healthy discipline for life.
9. Drink plenty of fluids	Drinking is a way to reduce the density of the gastric opening, thereby encouraging the circulation of air in the stomach.	Don't drink any milk if you are lactose-intolerant (use lactose-free formulas such as Lacteeze or Lactaid).
10. Apply warmth	Apply a hot "Magic Bag" on stomach, or take a hot bath.	Helps relax the entire digestive system. Makes it easier to release gas.
11. Dance	Similar to the "Technique Nadeau", dancing involves movements that promote gas circulation.	Helps rediscover the joy of the body. Encourages socialization.
12. Walk	Walk long enough to feel the rising of gases.	The abdomen should be relaxed and the intestines should be free to move during walk. Helps ascertain the extent of self-restraint.

13. Practise violent sports	Running, playing soccer, basket-ball, badminton, wrestling, judo, karate, boxing, etc., stirs and jiggles the body quite a bit.	Those who practice these sports often need their exercise "to feel better." Avoid overexertion.
14. Avoid holding it in as much as you can	Go to the bathroom, belch and fart as soon as you feel the need. You can even anticipate the need before you leave the house, or seize the opportunity to release yourself when you come across a restroom in a public place.	Avoid generating lasting stress to prevent gas build-up, sphincter contractions and excessive nervous tension.

RELEASING GAS FROM THE LARGE INTESTINE

The woman, a slave to prejudice, has never known the benefits of breaking wind (fart). For the past twelve years, an unhappy victim of her disease and of medicine, she had exhausted all remedies. Finally, enlightened about the usefulness of breaking wind, she farts freely and frequently. From that point on, no more pain, she is perfectly healthy.

Éloge du pet

EVACUATING THE DIGESTIVE SYSTEM

After practising for several months it becomes easier to identify the area of the digestive track that is affected by gas. It helps to adjust treatment, evaluate my condition, assess what I've accumulated over time, what I've gulped down diet-wise or socially, and to what extent I've let my body take charge of everything. It can also help determine how much improvement I can achieve by expelling gas from every part of my digestive track. This section details this process.

• The oesophagus

A faint, hoarse voice, a suffocating feeling, pain felt near the heart without there being cardiac or circulatory problems, pharyngitis, laryngitis, even asthma can be caused by air in the oesophagus. Hopefully, it takes only a few minutes to release it. Usually, it's merely the tip of the iceberg even though they can be very painful (a burning sensation) or dangerous (laryngitis, asthma, etc.). Gas in the oesophagus often signals – as in my case – a considerable quantity of gas throughout the digestive track. It is also possible that, in addition to the symptoms already described, to suffer from indigestion, diffuse back or intestinal pain, vagal fainting, which I so often experienced. Although epigastric symptoms can often be alleviated, they tend to reoccur as the gas moves up from the stomach into the oesophagus as internal pressure in upper digestive track equilibrates (fluid mechanics). You therefore have to keep burping.

After this, all the symptoms described relating to gas in the oesophagus will disappear, except when there is inflammation. This inflammation will be more easily treated if gases are evacuated regularly. Over time my voice remains clear and I no longer suffer from laryngitis at least once a year as I did in the past. I was invariably put on antibiotics, but since I've been belching systematically I no longer get infections or suffer from inflammatory disorders of the oesophagus. No more antibiotics. Moreover, once the oesophagus is cleared and the thoracic pain is eliminated, breathing becomes easier.

• The upper part of the stomach

Burning, cramps, loss of appetite, back pain behind the diaphragm are often caused by gases lodged in the upper part of the stomach. I generally need to belch for a half hour to evacuate them. However, here again relief is temporary and the pain is likely to return with the rising of air from the bottom of the stomach. In this area, gas can also block the upper part of the large intestine. Before this area is cleared, however, you may experience pain across the top part of your abdomen. It is very important, therefore, to evacuate this area, including the upper left part of the stomach, in order to restore circulation in the large intestine.

Once the oesophagus and the top part of the abdomen have been evacuated, you should be comfortable enough to do regular work. So, within three quarters of an hour (even less when the technique is well mastered), you can go from an extremely uncomfortable condition, like during a heartburn, to one comfortable enough for you to function. However, to really benefit from the gas evacuation exercises, you must be persistent.

• The middle part of the stomach

When the mid-section of the stomach is full of air I can feel a void, I'm hungry even after a meal, I feel bloated, my digestion is slowed down and I sometimes get hiccups. Back pain can also occur intermittently. I can even have kidney problems, water retention, headaches... or to urinate repeatedly late in the day. Every week I used to suffer from migraines lasting for days. They disappeared when the mid-section of my stomach was cleared up. Nowadays I rarely suffer from migraines, and fortunately I know what to do when it happens. Another effect of gas in that area is light sleep. This is a cause of fatigue.

Except for indirect pain such as backache and migraine, gas in the middle of the stomach is not as painful as when the gas is trapped higher up. The pain is not as localized; I just feel discomfort.

It takes at least an hour to clear this part of the stomach properly, and when there is bloating in that area it is more difficult to evacuate the gas. The whole arsenal of techniques is then needed (keeping hydrated, massaging the abdomen from all positions, pushing – bearing down –, applying warmth, rocking back and forth, etc.).

The rising of gas from that area can happen suddenly and be violent and painful, as hiccups can be.

Once the gas is evacuated the body and functions run smoothly, there is a feeling of well-being and deep breathing becomes easier. The back pain and migraines have disappeared, kidney functions have been restored, and with movement the flatulence goes away. Sleep is also greatly improved.

From a mental standpoint I become more available and my personality is more integrated. It is easier for me to act and think multi-dimensionally, as opposed to being paralysed by "intestinal conflicts". I no longer blunder. However, there is still room for improvement.

• The lower part of the stomach

Finally, the bottom of the stomach! When filled with air it makes you feel that your digestion is bogged down. Gas gets knotted with the lower part of the large intestine, bringing the circulation of intestinal gas at a standstill. I feel that it is in that specific area that the vicious circle of digestive problems originate. When gas sits at the bottom of the stomach it tends to lock in the large intestine and accumulate throughout the digestive track, which in turn puts pressure on the large intestine, etc. Total release "begins" with the evacuation of the bottom of the stomach. At that particular level I can feel the presence of gas in two places: behind the navel and at the bottom left, along the lower part of the large intestine. I need fifteen minutes more to clear this part of the stomach.

Here again the pain is not as spectacular but it is very treacherous. The consequences of letting gas sit at the bottom of the stomach are numerous and sometimes surprising: poor leg circulation, pinched sciatic nerve, migraines, indigestion, and faintness. To these pains I could add a depressed mood, which includes loss of enjoyment and even fear of motion, added to the feeling that the digestive system is totally stagnant.

In that case, the best results are obtained by bearing down, simulating defecation, vigorously massaging the lower abdomen, and taking deep breaths while loosening up the lower abdomen as much as possible. However, I cannot release that area if the upper part of the stomach has not already been cleared of gas. Since the stomach is very flexible at that point, I can go ahead enthusiastically and massage the abdomen extensively without feeling any pain at all, which I would be unable to do if my stomach was filled with air. The rising of the gas, even if it is sometimes spectacular, is not really painful.

When this area has been cleared I recover an outstanding quality of sleep. But first, the gas in the large intestine has to be evacuated, which can then be done naturally and rapidly. On the other hand, following a shock, or when there is persistent anxiety, ringing in the ears or intense muscular tension, the sleep deprivation tends to persist. To eliminate these symptoms, relaxation must come into play (see below).

In general, however, the pain disappears; I am at peace and even joyful! I am grateful to be alive since I now have this feeling of well-being! That's what I call my "normal state", a place where I can be myself, one that I almost never knew before the age of 35.

Even when I had my sciatic attacks, which I experienced in the 1990s following a double-disk hernia, the pain and inflammation abated after air was evacuated from my digestive track.

I also get my normal appetite back. I even feel that I can eat anything. Generally, my quality of life and sleeping habits persist for several days. If I accumulated fatigue by working at releasing gas for over two hours during the night, I can easily recuperate on the following nights. After three or four days, however, my digestive system begins storing up air again even if I've been eating well. So I go back to doing my exercises.

• The lower colon

Poor digestion (a knot in the pit of the stomach), slow kidneys, nocturnal emissions, sciatic nerve problems, colitis, diarrhoea, cold feet, dizziness, migraines, ringing in the ears can all be caused by gas accumulating in the rectum or lower colon. The most obvious symptoms include nocturnal emissions and leg cramps, especially in the calves. What we can do is bear down a little to feel the need to fart, which will then help get rid of the nocturnal emissions and the cramps. A frequent need to urinate can also occur, but without relieving ourselves completely.

Even after getting rid of a large quantity of air in the stomach, the large intestine may still be blocked. I start belching again to clear the gas at the bottom of the stomach, which I possibly thought had been completely removed. In such a case, the movement of gas in the large intestine is restored.

It is interesting to note that, once this is done, I get relief from the cramps and discomfort, and I sometimes get the impression that the cramps and discomfort can even vanish within a few minutes. This relief can last from a day to a week.

Once the flatulence is gone, all symptoms disappear. Moreover, my feces have a consistency that is neither too hard nor too soft, and I am very regular. When I do my exercises regularly I never experience diarrhoea or constipation. I never suffer from nausea, ringing in the ears, migraine or indigestion. Obviously I no longer suffer from vagal shock and I feel more comfortable in my social interactions: goodbye internal conflicts.

• The upper part of the colon

Shortness of breath, back pain, poor blood circulation, a feeling of being blocked are often caused by gas in the large intestine. The above-mentioned techniques relating to the lower colon also work for the upper colon. Once I get my lower colon evacuated, I am always surprised at how the gas from the upper colon can then move freely and painlessly. This also happens with the gas lodged in the large intestine on the right side of the abdomen. Generally, I get the impression that the gas doesn't accumulate as much in that area, compared with the gas that accumulates in the left part of the intestine. Once the gas from the lower colon has been evacuated I rest on my stomach for a little while. This position seems to help the movement of the gas located in the upper part of the colon.

Gas build-up can result from strong emotions that are repressed such as sorrow, fear (a jolt) and anger. As I mentioned, when people are aggressive, highly emotional or unpleasant I feel my large intestine tensing up. Psychologically, I feel that evacuating the gas from the higher part of the intestine helps me regain my ability to form social relationships. I feel that I am no longer frightened, no longer stuck.

When the evacuation is almost completed and very little gas remains, this is the best time for me to experience repressed emotions and ask myself what could have caused them, or what created this heavier gas accumulation or a higher tension that usual. It is also a time when I try to understand what is wrong, to make a good resolution, to pray. I finally understood, in fact, that as long as gas was still trapped in my digestive system I was not totally available and that I was not calm enough to create an effective inner dialogue. Otherwise I tend to run in circles, or my reflection is not integrative.

When I come across a word or event that may have been repressed on that day or in the last few days, generally, I feel a great thrill. It is as if my inner child started dancing with joy because I finally managed to accept reality and no longer held back. That inner child will no longer have to be responsible for everything, to cheat and cause me to somatise. I'm always grateful when this happens. It makes me feel free. I no longer need to watch myself in order not to blunder. I am no longer a threat to myself and others, and I do not experience any discomfort for a few days.

After I have experienced total release, I am greatly impressed by the difference between my personalities when I am filled with gas, and after I've evacuated all the gas. When life becomes difficult, shaky, I think about how I feel or what my decision would be if I was not "gassed up" and it helps me behave more appropriately. It is then easier for me to let go. But this is not done easily or automatically. In fact, when I experience a symptom that tells me I am full of air, I tend to be very careful, in my social relationships as well as in my physical activities, even if it means isolating me. When I was full of gas I blundered easily, even systematically, and risked hurting myself. So I often make an appointment with myself so to speak, that is, I plan a good evacuation session in the next few hours, or during the following night.

Paradoxically, I discovered that I could make use of the gas accumulated in the large intestine... to make myself dream. Anyway, in my case recurrent nightmares are a symptom of heavy gas accumulation. Sometimes I let the gas remain in my large intestine to help resolve a situation that I feel is deadlocked, when the efforts or attributes of my inner self are unable to get results. I may even concoct a meal with beans and lentils (the food of some African sorcerers). I retain or generate these gases because I know that they will make me dream. When I wake up I take stock of the situation. After I've found a more "creative" solution I expel the remaining gas and... sleep on it.

This allows me to focus on releasing nervous tension. I often alternate the release of gas and the release of nervous tension. Relaxing nervous tension facilitates the movement of gas and alleviates the pain caused by gas. Concurrently, it is difficult to alleviate nervous tension if there is a strong presence of gas.

Farts and belches are a recipe for good health!
Provencal saying

GETTING RID OF NERVOUS TENSION

I see nervous tension as an organic crisis, a world in itself, another dimension. Nervous tension has its own rules and cycles. According to me, when someone suffers from FDDs there is always diffuse tension and pain, which different people express differently. Tension and pain wander around in the body and systematically attack our weakest areas, or the ones we control the least.

I feel that we have a "natural rheostat" that helps us retain or reduce our perception of tension and pain. However, we can learn to use this rheostat to give these perceptions free rein, allow them to reach their full expression.

The basic principle I use to release nervous tension and pain is very simple: it involves directing excess nervous impulses to the point of fatigue. The concept of fatigue I use here is different from general fatigue, or the fatigue we feel when we are sleep deprived. I compare it to muscular fatigue. The stronger a muscle's contraction is, the more rapidly it will tire itself out. It is fortunate that the message sent by nervous tension has the same properties. The more I let the nervous tension come out, the easier it is to make it disappear. In fact, it is as if the tension was the expression of a deep discomfort. The more we let this discomfort express itself, the faster the tension it causes can be relieved.

I was introduced to relaxation techniques through transcendental meditation training. Unfortunately, I found this technique rather ineffective. So I tried to adapt the technique by lying on my back instead of sitting down, since I often felt like dozing off. During training we were told that when we felt like dozing off we should lie down and let it go. Although it wasn't as effective as meditation, it is what we needed most at that point.

As with meditation, we need a quiet place where we can be totally relaxed. In the past, when I practised meditation, I often started at the slightest noise, all the more reason to find a quiet spot for this exercise. Gas, dreams (remembering long-forgotten shocks the body still recalls) also often made me jump, and even triggered anxiety attacks. To quiet down and reassure myself I do my exercises with music I am familiar with (to avoid surprises), using my headphones. That way I can relax much more easily.

First, I slow down my respiratory rhythm as much as possible, making sure it doesn't become unbearable. I also reduce my air intake with each breath. If my cardiac rhythm accelerates, or if I feel the need to draw in a deep breath, I take it as a sign that I am not inhaling enough air. So I take a deep breath without overdoing it. I keep the air in for awhile before exhaling. Then, I slow down my respiratory rhythm once again, and reduce my air intake.

A sensation of stiffness in the body, or the impression that movement would be difficult follows, as in REM sleep. It is at this point that the nervous impulses take over. I then focus on the nervous tension, letting it express itself as much as possible instead of holding on to it, while continuing the breathing exercises. It is as if I was putting my hand on the rheostat which controls the sensations of pain and tension; as if I was increasing the tension running through my nervous system.

Then, I allow all the nervous impulses to increase, as well as all the symptoms. If I find that my body tries to hold on to the pain or tension, I regain my self-control. But as soon as I feel I can resume the exercise I repeat the procedure, allowing all the tensions and symptoms to increase. I remain well focused to make sure the tension remains at its peak for as long as possible. Sometimes this requires quite a bit of concentration. The natural tendency to hold back and regain self-control when one feels tension or pain can become insistent. But with experience, I try not to regain my self-control to release as much tension as possible in the shortest time possible. This method required several year of practice on my part.

When I first started this exercise I focused on the most obvious symptoms (cramps, migraine, eye pain, painful muscular tension, etc.). I used to let the tension rise in that particular spot until it got to be almost unbearable, but not to the point of having anxiety attacks, cramps or excessive pain. If this happened, the same as with nervous tension, I regained my self-control, and once I felt comfortable, I resumed the exercise. I could experience several crises in a row. There came a time when I couldn't trigger the crises as the excess tension eliminated itself. Even with a good control of the rheostat, there came a time when I could no longer magnify the message of tension and pain. The exercise then came to an end... for that part of the body I had been focusing on. I suggest that you begin with this exercise because you will need lots of practice before you can feel sufficiently safe to let all the symptoms increase simultaneously. On the other hand, when I feel very tense I go back to this method.

This is a method that can bring about anxiety attacks (I'll deal with this later). Once the attacks have been eliminated, and I feel I can get back to the nervous tension release exercises, I pick up again where I left off by focusing on the most obvious symptom and, letting it express itself, by magnifying it as much as possible. Once the heaviest symptom has been eliminated or substantially reduced, that is, once I find myself unable to magnify the message of tension or symptom, I proceed to the next one, the one that is the most easy to define in the body. I am always surprised of the extent to which a symptom I had previously focused on, one that had been had eliminated, could hide other symptoms.

After a while it becomes impossible to maintain the sensation or the nervous tension that causes the symptoms. The mechanism supporting the tension tires itself out, which brings on general relaxation. The entire process needs to be set in motion again until the excess nervous tension can hardly be felt at all. This is how I succeed in eliminating excess nervous tension. At first I did the exercise for at least 45 minutes, since it was often after only thirty minutes or so that I could feel the maximum tension.

When I try to release the nervous tension, it often happened – as in all forms of meditation – that images run through my head. I let them pass and then erase them. In fact, I use the blackboard technique. What you do is deposit the ideas on the board and make them disappear with an imaginary eraser. If they come back, they get erased again until I can focus on the part of the body that feels the most tension, and then increase the tension as much as possible.

If I can't manage it, I then try to think about something else, create a diversion, and I go back to doing the exercise. During an important attack of gas, images can jostle each other at a furious pace (this can happen when you have insomnia, for instance). You have to make sure that a great deal of gas is evacuated before resuming the nervous tension evacuation exercise. In my case, it is also a sign that I will need a long time, almost two hours, to totally get rid of the gas and nervous tension. If I don't spend as much time on the exercise I cannot go back to sleep, or I will have a restless sleep.

I do not recommend beginning the nervous tension evacuation exercises when a great deal of gas is present. It would then be almost impossible to relax anyway. I suggest that you evacuate about half the gas present in the stomach before loosening up or starting the relaxation technique. Afterwards it will be easier to make the gas circulate more thoroughly.

These past few years I have been in the habit of taking naps in the afternoon, during which I do the nervous tension evacuation technique almost exclusively. I also practice on week-ends, during the summer vacations and during the Holidays. For several years I asked that my salary be lowered so that I could add a week to my vacation every four months. Since I tend to take on too much, I could use that extra time to recharge my batteries. When I am on vacation for several weeks in a row, after ten days or thereabouts I don't feel as much need, or as many benefits, from doing the exercise. Sometimes I do the technique on Sunday morning when I sleep in. I find that this is when it is the most effective. Even after only a few minutes I feel more deeply relaxed than at any other time. I experience a salutary sluggishness that can last almost all day.

Since three years my job gained in complexity and in wage, so I came back full time in order to get the financial margin to be able to publish this version. It ended up with too much stress and conflicts at work so I left writing on this book for many months. Amazingly enough it is that stress that forced me to work on it again. I became zealous on my exercise routine and went back to reading to complete this book, since, at least, that's one of my way to be the boss in part of my life. That also helped me to pass from exercising for treatment to exercising for prevention of the pain. To do so, I changed my routine. I than belch half an hour everyday at evening to get good sleep, and I belch again for no more than 15 minutes around five in the morning, because I found that's the most effective time of the day to relieve quickly and without pain the most gazes in my system. I than can fall asleep again. I do try also to wake up later in the morning in order to have time to perform few minutes of my relaxation technique and the Dr Servan-Schreiber's heart coherence technique (see below). By doing so, the quality of my sleep improved greatly, and since I than wake up empty of gas and joyful in the morning, I do feel much better for my day of work.

Many outward signs that stem from excess nervous tension can be treated by my relaxation technique. Twitches, palpitations, kidney blockage, headaches, eye tension, ringing in the ears, etc., can be reduced or eliminated. However, for my symptoms to disappear completely it took me several months, even years, of daily practice (approximately an hour each day, or each night). What you need, therefore, is to get enough practice. I should emphasize that these symptoms are the body's attempt to rid itself of excess nervousness or stress. Therefore, it can take considerable time to correct the situation.

RELEASING THE PAIN

In my view, the pain and the symptoms are often the outward sign of nervous tension. This is why, when I perform the relaxation technique, I concentrate on the most obvious symptom, which I exaggerate to its point of fatigue. Then the tension decreases, and the pain along with it. When I was undergoing psychoanalysis I became aware that every one of my blockages had to do with a part of my body that felt tension and pain. The "suspended pain", as I call it, ultimately affects my personality, my ability to accept the world and its events, to adjust, to be self-assertive. Following my philosophical training I got into the habit of questioning the logic of that system. For example, I realized that when muscular tension is pushed to its limit, the muscles become exhausted. After a few years of psychoanalysis I was able to identify several symptoms of fibromyalgia. As the tension built up, my body was growing weaker and weaker.

Fortunately, the nervous tension evacuation technique, as I practise it, gets rid of the tension lodged in every part of the body. The tension that used to be located in those specific areas has been reduced, and so have the pain and the tension points (fibromyalgia). Moreover, some of the pain such as muscle pain or anxiety responds especially well to the release of nervous tension. The pain often varies; spectacularly increasing with disease, emotional events or without any apparent reason, but it can also disappear after a good night sleep, or leave as mysteriously as it came.

Over time, the relaxation technique systematically reduces the incidence of pain. For example, I couldn't practise any sport at thirty but now, as I am passed fifty, I am particularly active, even cross country skiing 8 kilometres many days a week to go to work on winter. Practising sports used to get me all stirred up. Invariably, I ended up suffering from stomach or back pain, and therefore had to cut down activities. Naturally, I was unaware of the benefits of exercise in combination with the release of gas and nervous tension.

A deep relaxation technique can help reduce tension which the nervous system cannot eliminate through sleep. In fact, I feel that the nervous tension and pain associated with FDDs symptoms are not adequately relieved by sleep. With the nervous tension release exercise, I manage it much more efficiently. One of the FDDs symptoms is visceral hypersensitivity. When I am doing the exercise I no longer feel the pain, even when there's still gas in my digestive system. I feel that the practise of a good relaxation technique is crucial to recovering a condition I would describe as normal.

This technique is very effective for anguish and anxiety attacks. When I have an anxiety attack I deal with it as I would for the symptoms that are easiest to locate. I increase the sensation of this symptom; I let myself feel this sensation as strongly and for as long as possible to eliminate all the nervous tension underlying it. Since I have good control of the internal rheostat, I can repeat the exercise. After doing it two or three times, the nervous tension release is impressive. This exercise easily eliminates the anxiety lying under the surface when I am full of gas. It also facilitates the evacuation of the gas ounce I pursue my relaxation technique up to decontracting my entire digestive track.

The tension accumulated around the eyes is often among the most obvious symptoms to come out during the exercise. It took me years before I let myself feel this tension around the eyes. It is particularly painful and causes a small anxiety attack almost every time. I was afraid of feeling too much pain to let myself go. However, the nervous rush I set loose when I focus on my eyes is significant. It is better to resort to this technique towards the end of the nervous tension evacuation exercise, which usually happens after three quarters of an hour. These days, since my general tension level is much lower, thanks to regular exercise sessions, this is where I begin my relaxation exercises. The degree of tension felt is an indication of the underlying tension. It tells me how long I should do the exercise to eliminate enough tension for me to go to sleep, or how long I should practice the gas evacuation exercises effectively.

During a migraine it is also possible to produce peaks of pain which, in this case also, will allow for a significant discharge of tension. These attacks can be magnified until they are eventually impossible to generate. What follows is an extraordinary feeling of relaxation. This technique can be used in the case of insomnia, to restore sleep quality. However, migraines require the combined practice of both gas and nervous tension evacuation techniques. Usually I need between an hour and an hour and a half of combined evacuation exercises to transform a migraine into a mild headache that lets me function normally.

However, I don't think that could work for all types of migraines, such as the migraine caused by high blood pressure, or inflammation.

For several years I suffered intermittently from eye tics. I realized that releasing gas sometimes made the tics completely disappear. I almost never suffer from them any longer, but when it happens I know that I have a great deal of air trapped in my digestive track. All I need is an hour of combined exercises to eliminate them.

It is the same with the ringing in the ears. God knows how much it can be detrimental to the quality of life. I discovered that I could get rid of this ringing every time I completely evacuated the gas and nervous tension. In my case, the ringing in the ears, contrary to the tics, responds very well to the virtual rheostat exercise. It is easy to exaggerate this symptom, maintain it at that level for a long time and finally, eliminate it to eventually reach a point where you can't produce it any more. The disappearance of the ringing is a sign that a great tension has finally been released. However, it takes me at least two hours of combined exercises to get rid of it.

Muscular tension, especially in the abdominal muscles, forearms and neck, also responds well to the rheostat. Besides, it took me years of practice to permanently relax my abdominals (see chapter on Pierre Pallardy below). Once this was done, once this curtain had been lifted, I discovered that this tension masked several FDDs symptoms. It is as if a solid lid had been put on everything that was simmering inside. It is my impression that the persistent contraction of these muscles reflects my inability to let go, my wish to remain in control and not feel the pain I feel in my body.

However, I never succeeded in practising the rheostat using my back muscles, or lumbar or leg muscles. However, since these muscles respond well to stretching, I added stretching exercises to my routines.

Why weren't these techniques developed and made available in the past? The answer is relatively simple: to loosen up and release nervous tension is anything but pleasant, especially at first. It's not that interesting to relive a bad experience. Try to convince somebody that, in order to feel better, they must go through a painful loosening up at least twenty times in a row. The release of nervous tension can also trigger anxiety attacks that can be particularly unpleasant.

At this point, I wish to emphasize the need to get to grips with the pain level, because the pain can be strong and repetitive during the release of nervous tension, especially at the stage of the exaggeration of symptoms. We must learn to "direct" the pain. For example, if you have a cramp it is more painful to feel it and visualise the path it must follow to find an exit, than to try and hold it in. But the exacerbation of the pain is short-lived compared to when you try to hold it in, which may cause the original pain to return. Release cannot be achieved without pain, without us becoming aware of that pain and deciding to accept it. We have to make room for it. We must be in good shape to let in this further pain that is ultimately good for us.

We must go from a condition where the pain is feared and avoided to one where it becomes a valuable ally, an enlightener. Without becoming a masochist, it can be said that we have to suffer to be well.

During difficult times, the natural tendency to avoid pain causes us to neglect ourselves. There is always a high risk of going back to our former state of being stuck, of regressing. It is only through our sustained efforts, through regular self-analysis that progress can be achieved.

Managing the pain, letting it take over the space we allow it to take, and through it assert ourselves in our relationship with the pain, forces us to develop techniques that we can use to manage its excesses. It is crucial not to give up. When the pain reaches a peak during a relaxation session we can, as I sometimes do, repeat a mantra, pray to find the courage to keep it up and maintain the pain at that level for as long as we can. We could imagine that a guardian angel, a therapist, a kindly paternal or maternal representation or a friend takes us by the hand. When I have a bout of eye pain I, for example, recite the "Our Father" while I wait for it to go away. Usually, this is sufficient.

As I was progressing in my analysis I discovered that every time a pain finally faded, a new one took over. The pain, the tension, the hysteria moved around. Every part of my body would reveal deep secrets, a repression I needed to relive and deal with in a different way. The painful events of the past are often repressed. We may have caused this repression, in part, consciously. Perhaps we told ourselves that a particular event was too difficult to handle, at the time we may have been unable to deal with it but had to go on living. In psychoanalysis, it is the memory of these small bits of consciousness that allow us to go back over the causes of our tension, of our dysfunction.

Working on these new discomforts can give us the impression that we are regressing, that we are now dealing with new pain we didn't have before. Why should we discover a new symptom when it took so much effort to get rid of the old one? It is especially important not to give up. We must believe that it is possible to reach the last of the symptoms.

Frequently, the same repressed emotions, or those the body had to come to terms with, create discomfort in the same regions of the body. I previously mentioned the connection between my anger and the contraction of the large intestine. In my case, stress is mainly handled by the stomach, and I sometimes feel that it stops functioning altogether. I may occasionally fell the need to be physically stuck in the same way as I get stuck psychologically, to restore balance. Therefore, releasing the gas and the nervous tension means agreeing to get unstuck psychologically, agreeing to change. It means taking care of my soul. Who would have imagined that we could take care of our souls in this way?

After several years of practice, while exercising some caution, it is even possible to treat obsessions or mania in this way, whether we are dealing with imaginary conflicts, internal anger, or phobias. Here too we need to find a quiet place and be by ourselves, to push symptoms to their limits, as with nervous tension, to go as far as possible while respecting the following condition: "delirium and the obsessions", regardless of their violence, must never control our actions and should never put us, or someone else, at risk. Letting the symptoms be pushed to the limit without commanding an action enables us to assess the unreal, dysfunctional nature of those symptoms... The good way to treat them is to "wear them out."

Table II Relaxation and Pain Relief Technique		
Stage	**Why**	**Remark**
Slow down the breathing	• slow down the metabolism • put ourselves in a state of REM consciousness	• if the cardiac rhythm accelerates, go back to breathing normally
Relax all systems	• reduce the holding in or fear of the pain • restore the movement of the gas and nervous energy	• the contraction, controlling attitude always returns
Release the most significant pain first	• let the pain reach the point of nervous fatigue • take your mind off the other pain • increase the relaxation	• if the pain becomes too intense or causes anxiety, regain your self-control • resume the relaxation
Wipe out ideas that come up, don't think twice about it	• let the body express itself instead of the mind • learn to put things into perspective	• Ideas that repeat themselves or occur in too quick a succession indicate a high level of physical and nervous tension or obsession
Relax sufficiently	• increase the effectiveness of therapies and other release activities • improve the quality of life	• the optimum release occurs after 30 minutes (you should therefore practice for at least 45 minutes)

Letting the anxiety express itself	• release a maximum of tension • de-dramatize the anxiety • learn to assume it • make it your ally	• consider anxiety as an intense, generalized symptom • if one attack is over, try to live out another one and so on, until it exhausts itself
Elevating your pain threshold	• release as much tension as possible in a short period of time • assess the general condition • learn to identify your psychosomatic responses	• avoid losing control (fit of hysterics, cramps) • the higher the threshold of pain, the quicker the tension is released
Increasing the pain of a symptom for as long as you can	• eliminate as much tension as possible • with time, eliminate the symptom • help decipher what is hidden behind the symptom (try to reach its limit)	• if you are unable to keep the pain at a high level, try to re-establish it several times before moving on to another symptom
Trying to practise all these steps at once	• master the technique • practising all these steps simultaneously becomes much less tedious • (I describe them separately for better understanding)	• it may take time before you find the best method in your case

Finally, as shown in the above table, let's see how we can combine several exercises. For example, when I do the relaxation exercises I can inflate my abdomen, rock gently back and forth and belch at the same time. Or, as I stretch while lying down on my right side I focus on the pain that is the most obvious, the pain around the eyes, for instance, then I can reduce my air intake, gently rock back and forth, and belch. These combination exercises accelerate the treatment. In just one hour I can explore the most obvious symptoms while relaxing, evacuating the gas trapped in my stomach and large intestine, rocking back and forth while I get stirred up, changing positions often, while breathing deeply and reducing my air intake alternately. Performing the exercises one at a time is boring, and it may take two or three times longer to achieve convincing results that way. What I need, therefore, is about an hour to free myself from most FDDs-related symptoms in a natural way, without medication.

THE RELIEF

The presence of gas brings about tension in the muscular and nervous systems. A deep release occurs following the evacuation exercises. It is an ideal time, if we don't fall back to sleep or resume the activities we previously gave up, to question ourselves, let ourselves live out the emotions that may have caused our condition. We can make an inventory of recent events and try to remember if the emotions they triggered are similar to those experienced during childhood. It is also a good time for analysis.

We could ask ourselves: "Do I still feel physical pain or frustration, but also pleasures, dreams to fulfil?" A total release can give us a few hours, sometimes a few days' break during which we can feel normal, be in control and live our lives as we would like to.

Naturally, we could be content and go no further: I feel better, so I'll take advantage of that feeling. However, it is better to discipline ourselves, question ourselves to ensure that our overall health condition is evolving positively, assess the possibility of becoming an optimist towards life again. Day-to-day problems can be seen in a totally different light when we have completely evacuated the gas, the excess nervous tension and the pain.

One thing is certain, after the gas and nervous tension are gone; the quality of sleep improves greatly. If sleep doesn't come easily it's probably because there hasn't been a total release, or the anxiety level is still high. Naturally, if we almost never succeed in getting a good night's sleep, the thing to do is see a doctor. Normally, a night of improved sleep compensates for the fatigue built up while we were dealing with our symptoms, which I often do during the night. Generally, I experience a deep, prolonged sleep on the night following the one during which I exercised extensively.

When there is diarrhoea, disruptions, or during therapy, total release lasts only for a day. When conditions improve, the release may last up to a week. In my case, the accumulation of gas doesn't stop.

Evacuating gas and excess nervous tension therefore provides an opportunity to express ourselves with a great deal more satisfaction. In fact, a so-called "normal" condition helps make me more available. We have to listen to our inner child, to integrate it, to become no longer victim of its excesses. Freeing an inner space can be compared to a "spring cleaning", as we say in Quebec. We can then make new friends, get in touch with old acquaintances and develop mutually satisfying relationships.

WHAT WE CAN EXPECT FROM IT AND THE LIMITATIONS

• To exist

According to Dr Dufour, in *Les tremblements intérieurs* (p. 38): "There is an elementary and essential rule: nobody but ourselves can give us the right to exist. To exist means to live out our emotions, to follow our desires. Nobody truly exists if they do not allow themselves to do so". In a way, the exercises I propose are part of the right to exist that I bestow upon myself.

- ## It is not a cure (does not replace medicine)

The relaxation and gas evacuation techniques do not cure FDDs. However, I can safely say that, the release of gas helps relax the stomach and stimulate the movement of the gastric bowl. I can say that, after the gas has been evacuated, I feel cured temporarily. It is not a complete cure, but with practice I've felt that the motility has gradually improved, and so has the resilience of the nervous system.

- ## We should stick with it and do it often

This temporary feeling of well-being only returns when the exercises, especially those that concern gas, are repeated. In my case, three days elapse, at the most, before I need to clear my system once again. As the days go by, I feel that my quality of life, my well-being and my availability are declining. At that point, the approach that consists in integrating the technique into daily activities whenever possible is very useful.

When experiencing a period of stress or dietary neglect, I increase the pace and intensity of the treatment. Stress slows down digestion and promotes the accumulation of gas, so that I have to be on the watch for signs of stress and be ready to practice my exercises zealously, if necessary. During periods of stress it is more difficult to increase our "regularity." It takes a strong dose of discipline and courage to carry on and make it through. It is obviously easier to do nothing and feel awful.

It is often difficult to maintain healthy eating habits. However, I should make the effort to maintain a balanced diet. Naturally, as I begin to feel better, I can reward myself with small pleasures, while avoiding excesses. I often give myself a treat and then, when zeal comes into play everything eventually turns out all right.

One of my new habits is to exercise even if I feel well. It amazes me how many gas could be left in my digestive track even if I don't feel bad. Obviously, I feel even much better afterward. As I said before, gas could build up naturally without stress, but if I let them in, that will become painful and stressful. So driving them out before I could even feel bad is a good way to feel as if I am not having IBS.

- **Discomfort, at first**

The first time a pocket of gas is released from the bottom of the stomach, we may remain with a feeling of shock and not want to relive this experience. This indeed can have a surprising even painful. Moreover, as we release gas and the pain from the stomach, new discomforts can be revealed. We should not throw in the towel when facing a new symptom, even if it is persistent. When we carry on with the practise, adapting it to the new symptoms, it is possible to tone them down and, after some time has passed, move on to something else.

An improvement of the gastric system's condition also reveals the solitary or isolated state in which we often find ourselves in order to make life more bearable. When we realize this, we may feel a deep sadness. Our joy returns as our well-being improves, as we renew pleasurable relationships and develop new ones. Also, with practice, especially relaxation, gas release from the bottom of the stomach can become much less painful.

- **Overcoming the fear of being physically active, of inner movement**

Freeing ourselves from gas, nervous tension and pain can stir us up. It is particularly difficult to transcend the fear of pain related to this internal stirring. Getting stirred up can even provokes anxiety, especially at first. We can console ourselves by realizing that our past anxiety attacks are not likely to come back. It is through relaxation at first, then by our own efforts and will that we can start moving, that we generate and accept internal movement so that we can reap the rewards that come our way. But, at least, we get to decide how much is too much, and why, and we're the ones who will ultimately feel better. It is at this point that we share in what I call "the Peter Pan adventure." We can do something for ourselves, by treating FDDs.

• Variations (really falling ill, gastro, etc.)

Even if we regularly do the release exercises we can still fall ill occasionally or have more symptoms than usual. Following a severe stress, accumulated fatigue or even a bout of flu, our perception and our efforts to recover may be heightened. Therefore, we should try to find out if our feeling of discomfort occurs when we are in a normal state of health. We may be anxious when the discomfort we experience is more pronounced than usual. If this occurs during an illness, then we should treat that illness. We should be aware that in this case we may experience more discomfort and anxiety than usual. Paradoxically, following an illness we may be glad to recover our usual symptoms. This often happens with spring gastro, for instance.

Another possibility is that our discomfort is the result of an improvement of our overall condition. For example, when we feel relaxed towards the end of a vacation, a significant amount of gas or anxiety may enter the picture. This occurs with migraine sufferers. They often have an attack during the week-end, that is to say, after they've been resting. Anxiety is often expressed following a shock or a stressful period. The treatment must be continued even when we feel like giving up, or when we are unable to associate the symptoms with their causes.

• The feeling that something can be done to treat FDDs

One of the most important aspects of the practice of all the proposed exercises is what I call their "placebo effect". The feeling of well-being that results from the exercises is one thing, but to experience the reality of getting rid of the symptoms that seemed uncontrollable is particularly energizing. It can be a crucial step in getting relief from a depressive state that could eventually develop because of accumulated symptoms. In this context, Anglophones refer to *empowerment*. However, I should point out that my approach is not officially recognized as a procedure by modern medicine.

4 – Literature Review

A) – FUNCTIONAL DIGESTIVE DISORDERS (FDDs)

This chapter includes highlights from several texts on FDDs, which I consulted over the past fifteen years to add to the book's interest. The first part deals with the Rome criteria used by health care professionals to clarify and homogenise the description of the various disorders and their treatments. Later on, the main symptoms will be dealt with separately. Gas and flatulence, gastroesophageal reflux, asthma, constipation, diarrhoea, gastro, migraine, vagal fainting and haemorrhoids will then be discussed. Subsequently, several causes mentioned in literature will also be broached. We will discuss food allergies, monosodium glutamate, diverticulitis, *helicobacter pylori*, ulcers and anxiety. The connection between FDDs and inflammatory disease will also be brought up, to differentiate them and alleviate fears.

The assumption that another "brain" manages the entire digestive track and may be influenced or helped by our efforts will be discussed. The influence of the central nervous system and of former traumas, the psychosomatic angle, and depression, will also be reviewed. Finally, other types of exercises referred to in literature, as well as the more classic treatments such as the diet, will be summed up.

According to Drs Pierre Paré and Marc Bradette (*Le Clinicien*, vol. 11, n° 4, April 1996), FDDs physiopathology is composed of three elements: motility, visceral perception abnormalities, and psycho-social factors. The motility problems observed in the stomach, the colon, and occasionally the small intestine areas, generally consist of an abnormal myoelectric activity. In the case of functional dyspepsia (nervous stomach), the abnormalities involve digestive motility, irritable colon combined with diarrhoea, hypomotility and, in the case of irritable colon combined with constipation, hypermotility. To this should be added, a lowering of the visceral perception threshold, i.e., an increased feeling of pain when gas is present in the stomach, colon and small intestine.

Patients with FDDs (generally in combination with IBS) generally complain of extradigestive symptoms: tension headaches, backache, high blood pressure, urinary urgency, muscle pain consistent with fibromyalgia, non-coronary retrosternal pain, chronic fatigue, chronic pelvic pain, and in women, dyspareunia or pain during sexual intercourse, dysmenorrhoea or menstrual pain. In general, these patients tend to seek medical attention frequently. For example, about 60% of people with fibromyalgia also have IBS. According to several studies whose results are published in the brochure *Le SCI et vous, Mieux vivre avec le syndrome du côlon irritable* (IBS), Jouveinal inc., it was revealed that, out of a hundred patients who have IBS, all experienced abdominal pain, abdominal distension and alternating diarrhoea/constipation; 96 were in a constant lethargic state; 75 had back pain; 73, an early bloating sensation at mealtime; 66, excessive eructation; 62, nausea; 61, migraines; 56, urinary problems and 51, heartburn and dyspepsia. Other symptoms were also noted: skin dryness, pain in the thighs, bad breath, dizzy spells, and general discomfort.

According to Drs Paré and Bradette, no pharmacological breakthrough is likely to solve FDDs problems. The main therapeutic objective is therefore to relieve the symptoms, which cannot always be successfully controlled or eliminated. The intervention recommended is based on three different levels: a general approach, an approach specific to the predominant symptom, and a global approach (bio-psychosocial) in the case of stubborn patients.

The global approach consists in providing information and promoting the patient-doctor relationship. Doctors should reassure patients and make sure they understand that FDDs are a genuine pathological condition, let them know about its psychosocial and precipitating factors and its dietary and emotional influence factors. A good patient-doctor relationship reassures the patient, who may be less inclined to seek medical attention. Patient should be encouraged to examine emotional factors that could be at play in their disorder. This effort will yield better results than if they search for an isolated cause for their acute anxiety or stress.

A specific approach focusing on the predominant symptom (pharmacological therapy) is preferable if the symptoms are severe or stubborn. There is a strong placebo effect involved in the FDDs, so that medication is only recommended sporadically, or for short periods. In cases involving a nervous stomach, few studies conclude that medication has a positive effect. Randomized control group studies suggest that muscle relaxants and antidepressants can significantly improve abdominal pain. Clinical experience also suggests that antispasmodic medication is also helpful. For example, the book IBS for Dummies (p. 175) suggests that magnesium phosphate is an antispasmodic medicine that treats cramping of all muscle groups, including those that produce hiccups, leg cramps, writer's cramp, abdominal colic, heart pain, lung pain, and menstrual pain.

According to Dr Georges Ghattas (*Le Clinicien*, December 2003, p. 67), no algorithm is complex enough to take into account all the implications found in these words: "Doctor, I have abdominal pain!" To make the medical idiom more specific, researchers from the United States, Italy, Australia and Canada met in Rome, first in 1988 (Rome I), then in 2000 (Rome II), to propose a classification for FDDs (see Table I). This nomenclature was later validated by research. In the absence of scientific data, the consensus approach prevailed. Finally, in May 2006, the new FDDs diagnostic criteria, also called the Rome III criteria, were disclosed by a scientific committee stemming from the *Rome Foundation*, made up of over 100 world renowned experts, at the annual conference of the American Gastroenterological Association. FDDs affect all the organs of the digestive tract. Functional dyspepsia (nervous stomach), as well as IBS, are the most common and are defined by very specific criteria. This classification underscores the complexity of these disorders, which are made up of multiple, often similar, symptoms.

At first[8], we must distinguish between a symptom, which is something that you say is happening to you, and a sign, which is something objective that a doctor observes or finds on physical examination. With both, doctor investigates to diagnose a disease, syndrome, or condition. IBS is hard to diagnose since it is a syndrome and not a disease. On average, women consult three practitioners before being adequately diagnosed with IBS.

• **The Rome Criteria**

Here is a summary published by Pierre Poitras, gastroenterologist, in the journal of the *Association des maladies gastro-intestinales fonctionnelles* (AMGIF), *Du cœur au ventre*, on the Rome criteria. Dr Poitras kindly allowed me to publish a summary of this work. It includes, among other things, the medical treatment suggested for the most frequent ills and for IBS, including functional dyspepsia (nervous stomach).

---

[8]   IBS for Dummies, p. 123.

Table III	
Functional digestive disorder according to the Rome criteria	
A. OESOPHAGEAL DISORDER A.1 Bolus A.2 Rumination syndrome A.3 Chest pain presumably of oesophageal origin A.4 Functional (oesophageal) heartburn A.5 Functional dysphagia A.6 Unspecified functional oesophageal disorder	**B. GASTRO-DUODENAL DISORDER** B.1 Functional dyspepsia B.1a. ulcerous type B.1b. motor type B.1c. non specific type B.2 Aerophagia B.3 Functional vomiting
C. INTESTINAL DISORDER C.1 Irritable bowel syndrome C.2 Functional abdominal bloating C.3 Functional constipation C.4 Unspecified functional intestinal disorder	**D. FUNCTIONAL ABDOMINAL PAIN** D.1 Functional abdominal pain syndrome D.2 Unspecified functional abdominal pain
E. FUNCTIONAL DISORDER OF THE BILIARY TREE AND PANCREAS E.1 Gall bladder dysfunction E.2 Dysfunction of Oddi's sphincter	**F. ANORECTAL DISORDER** F.1 Functional fecal incontinence F.2 Functional anorectal pain F2a. levator syndrome F2b. proctalgia fugax F.3 Pelvic floor dyssynergia (anism)

This classification is meant to diagnose and provide physicians and gastroenterologists with treatment strategies based on the symptoms. Without this classification, the risks of faulty diagnoses and treatments would be higher.

Sick people often have more than one symptom. The same patient frequently presents digestive symptoms in the lower irritable bowel, and the higher abdominal discomforts of functional dyspepsia. There are also symptoms that shift from IBS to functional dyspepsia, or vice versa.

A – Chest pains of oesophageal origin (non cardiac)

The fairly frequent **chest pain presumably of oesophageal origin** (A.3) is a sudden, intense, intermittent pain occurring day or night, often oppressive and accompanied by a tightening or torsion of the thorax, which can irradiate to the jaw or the arm and can send a patient to the hospital, fearing a heart attack. This chest pain has to have occurred at least once a week for a period of three months during the previous six months. It cannot be accompanied by abdominal pain from other areas, and it is not relieved by defecation or the release of flatulence. The nitroglycerin used for heart attacks is sometimes effective in the case of oesophageal pain. Invariably cardiac tests turn out normal, as do the lungs and musculoskeletal tests. The oesophagus is identified by default as the source of this pain. Generally, diseases related to these cases are not life-threatening. However, in many cases there are few treatments available and the pain is persistent. In roughly half of the cases, gastroesophageal reflux, with or without inflammation of the oesophagus (oesophagitis) is present (see chapter on reflux). It can be treated by blocking (with Losec, Prevacid, Pantoloc and Nexium medications, for example) the acid secretion rising up from the stomach. Specific motor disorders – such as achalaxia or diffuse oesophageal spasms, sporadic spasms without an identifiable cause, or hypersensitivity of the oesophagus – are rarely diagnosed. As with other FDDs, oesophageal hypersensitivity heightens discomfort that would normally be tolerable or not felt.

Nitroglycerin has the capacity to relax muscular spasms of the oesophagus. Intestinal analgesics can reduce visceral sensitivity. Stress management occasionally helps. Functional chest pain does not develop into other more serious pathologies such as cancer.

Globus (A.1) is a sensation of spasm, of contraction or of a lump in the throat. A spasm of the upper muscle of the oesophagus has been documented in some people. The **rumination syndrome** (A.2) is rare. It is characterized by the regurgitation of undigested food, and its re-mastication. This process, a normal one for ruminants, is caused by an abnormal reflex, or a bad habit in humans. Biofeedback psychotherapy can be used to correct it. Biofeedback is non-invasive, has no side effects, and puts you in control. The average number of treatments for IBS is six to eight held over a three-month period. The National Institutes of Health shows about 75 to 80 percent reduction in symptoms of IBS[9]. **Functional (oesophageal) heartburn** (A.4) is a more common ailment causing chest discomfort in the form of a burning sensation similar to gastroesophageal reflux; however, no abnormal acid reflux is revealed upon investigation. It is highly likely that hypersensitivity makes acid reflux that would hardly be felt in normal circumstances, painful. Reducing normal acid secretion could help in these cases. **Functional dysphagia** (A.5) can be described as a difficulty in swallowing food, or a sensation of blockage during the transit of food along the oesophagus. Visceral hypersensitivity is often involved.

Functional oesophageal disorders are common and can be unsettling when they mimic cardiac problems, for example. They are often associated with other functional digestive problems such as dyspepsia or IBS.

B – Functional dyspepsia

Functional or non-ulcerous dyspepsia is the most common type of dyspepsia. According to the Digest study involving 1,036 Canadians, 21% of the respondents have this problem. Another Canadian study published in the Journal of Gastroenterology concludes that, in Canada, 29% of adults experience symptoms of dyspepsia at least once a week.

---

[9]   Ibid p. 227.

B1 – Functional dyspepsia: diagnostic criteria

Disorders that last at least twelve weeks – not necessarily consecutively – during the previous six months, with patients presenting any of the following symptoms:

1. Persistent or recurring pain or discomfort centered in the upper abdomen, premature sensation of burning or satiety;
2. No evidence of organic disease (following an investigation by gastroscopy, for example) that could explain the symptoms;
3. No evidence that the dyspepsia is relieved exclusively by defecation or is related to beginning changes in the frequency and form of the stools (no IBS).

For doctors, dyspepsia refers to a wide variety of symptoms, including epigastric pain, excessive eructation, abdominal bloating, indigestion, nausea and sometimes vomiting. Several factors play a role in dyspepsia: acidic secretion, inflammation of the stomach or duodenum, food intolerance, lifestyle, psychological factors, medication, *helicobacter pylori*, infections, etc. Over 80% of patients suffering from IBS also have symptoms suggesting functional dyspepsia (nervous stomach), whereas over one third of patients with functional dyspepsia present symptoms that suggest IBS.

Functional dyspepsia can be assessed by a gastric emptying test: 40% of cases show a delay in gastric emptying of solids or liquids. However, when prokinetics are prescribed to normalize gastric emptying, they fail to reduce the symptoms. That's why doctors rarely propose a gastric emptying test as a diagnostic tool. As in the case of IBS, visceral hypersensitivity and psychological problems are involved. Patients may consult for these reasons.

In the case of **ulcerous dyspepsia** (B.1a) the pain, centered in the upper abdomen (epigastric), can be reduced or increased by eating, and alleviated with antacids (Tums, Maalox, Zantac, Losec, etc.). As in the case of **motor dyspepsia** (B.1b), ulcerous dyspepsia is an unpleasant or uncomfortable epigastric sensation that is not painful but is sometimes characterized by or associated with an impression of fullness in the upper abdomen, bloating or nausea.

In the case of **ulcerous dyspepsia**, some tests help eliminate the possibility of gall bladder or pancreatic diseases which may produce similar symptoms. Medications used to treat ulcers, i.e., antacids (Rolaids, Tums, etc.), H2 blockers (Zantac, Pepcid, etc.) and proton pump inhibitors (Losec, Prevacid, Pantoloc, etc.) help control the pain. However, some people only find relief when given strong medication (double dosage) for extended periods (one to two weeks). If the hyposecretive treatments fail, medication acting on stomach sensitivity such as Elavil (amitriptyline), or antidepressants that are serotonin agents (Paxil, Celexa, Zoloft, Luvox, Prozac, etc.) can be used.

With motor dyspepsia, there may be problems of stomach relaxation or sensitivity. A "non relaxable", highly tonic stomach rapidly produces a sensation of fullness or excessive eating. An overly sensitive stomach leads to discomfort or pain that a "normal" individual only feels with considerably more distension.

The blocking of acid secretion reduces the amount of liquid (two litres a day) secreted by the stomach at mealtime. This reduces the stomach's swelling. To help contract a "lazy" stomach, medication that has a stimulating effect, such as metoclopramide (Maxeran), domperidone (Motilium) or tegaserode (Zelmac), can be used. A hypertensive stomach can be relaxed with antispasmodic medications (Bentylol), and a hypersensitive stomach with visceral analgesics such as amitriptyline or serotonin agents (Paxil, Celexa, etc.).

If the symptoms are resistant to the usual treatment, a low-dosage tricyclic antidepressant, or a serotonin recapture inhibitor, can be used to relieve the pain. However, few studies have shown their effectiveness.

It is suggested that non pharmacological means can also be used to relieve ulcerous or motor dyspepsia, including psychotherapy (behavioural, helping relationships or others). IBS symptoms are often chronic, interspersed with calm periods of various lengths. Therefore, we should not be surprised if we need to renew therapeutic interventions as time passes.

Functional vomiting (B.3) is cyclic, and occurs less than once a week. There has to be at least three episodes of this vomiting within a year, with no nausea or vomiting between episodes. The Rome III criteria also add chronic nausea as an IBS symptom. According to these criteria, in the previous six months, over a twelve-week period, this nausea can occur several times a week. However, the chronic nausea cannot be explained by vomiting or disease.

C – Intestinal disorders

C.1 Irritable Bowel Syndrome (IBS): diagnostic criteria
For at least twelve weeks – not necessarily consecutive – during the previous six months, a person must experience abdominal discomfort or pain that includes the following three characteristics:

1. the feeling of discomfort is relieved by defecation;
2. discomfort is related to a change in stool frequency;
3. discomfort is related to a change in the stools' form or appearance.

Other symptoms supporting the IBS diagnosis:
- abnormal stool frequency (more than three a day, or less than three a week);
- shape of stools is abnormal (hard, dry, too soft or liquid);
- abnormal stool transit (straining upon defecation, urgent defecation or sensation of incomplete emptying);
- passing of mucus;
- bloating or sensation of distended abdomen.

More often than most, people who suffer from IBS also have abdominal cramps, bloating, constipation or diarrhoea. The problem of stool frequency may be the result of intestinal hyperactivity or hypersensitivity. Excessive intestinal contractions tend to slow down the progression of the bolus leading to gas formation, therefore to resistance to the passage of the stool and consequently to cramps. For some, bloating is so important that their clothes have to be loosened. A sensation of incomplete emptying is sometimes felt. From a psychological point of view, patients may feel anxious, depressed, with low self-esteem, fear, guilt and anger. Non digestive symptoms include sleep anomalies, chronic back or pelvic pain, headaches, interstitial cystitis (pelvic pain with an urgent need to urinate), pain in the temporomandibular joint (face and head), and post-traumatic stress.

In Western countries it is estimated that between 10% and 15% of population suffer from digestive problems akin to IBS. Only 25% of those patients see their doctor about their complaint. They also count from 25% to 50% of gastroenterology consultations. Subjects who suffer from psychological factors (anxiety and somatisation) consult more for their pain than for intestinal problems.

The *IBS Self Help Group of Canada* (www.ibsgroup.org) has mandated the Ipso-Reid firm to survey 300 of its members, who guaranteed that they had been diagnosed with IBS in 2002. Over 85% of those surveyed considered that their symptoms were very unpleasant to extremely unpleasant, and that they negatively affected their work, their travels and their social activities. Forty-five percent of them felt IBS was detrimental to their quality of life. A number of studies suggest that quality of life of such patients compares with those suffering from depression, and is worse than those with type-2 diabetics or heart attack. Nearly half of the respondents experienced these symptoms daily, while 27% indicated that they happened two to three times a week. A third considered their symptoms to be serious.

Work can also affect IBS. Many people[10] surveyed by a questionnaire of Alimentary Pharmacology & Therapeutics Journal can trace the onset of their IBS to coincide with a new job, an increased workload, a change in staff or management, or a reduction in job satisfaction.

---

[10]   Ibid p. 252.

During the three months preceding the survey, the average number of work or school days lost as a result of IBS added up to 6, and 9.3 in the case of personal activities. Moreover, 12% of the respondents indicated that they had been or were currently on disability leave because of IBS.

According to Dr Pierre Paré, IBS is an invalidating disorder that weighs heavily on the Canadian health care system, and costs approximately eight hundred million dollars (some six hundred million Euros) a year. In the U.S., diagnosing and treating IBS may cost the healthcare system in excess of 29 billion dollars per year[11].

However, IBS is neither dangerous nor progressive, i.e., it does not put the patient's life at risk or develop into life threatening diseases such as cancer, Crohn's disease, etc. Although IBS involves chronic pain, most medical examinations (X-rays, endoscopy, etc.) reveal normal organs. The correction of the stool transit does not necessarily eliminate the pain. It is increasingly thought that this pain is the result of intestinal hypersensitivity. An experimentation led by Dr Poitras reveals that from 80% to 90% of patients suffering from IBS experience intestinal hypersensitivity. Subjects who have irritable bowels generally present a higher cutaneous perception level.

Depending on the case, doctors can prescribe antispasmodic medication, including antiacetylcholines (Bentylol, Levsin, etc.), anticalcic medication (Dicetel) and opiates (Modulon, Imodium) to reduce motility. To accelerate motility, the doctor may suggest adding fibres to the diet, using laxatives (magnesium, Colytel) or prokinetics (Motilium, Prepulsid, etc.). To reduce intestinal hypersensitivity, antidepressants that are serotonin capture inhibitors (Paxil, Prozac, Celexa, Luvox, Serzone, Efexor, etc.) or amitriptyline (Elavil) can be prescribed. Obviously, other approaches such as a better diet, psychotherapy, hypnosis, helpful relationships, progressive relaxation, etc., can also be helpful. According to the ***Association des maladies gastro-intestinales fonctionnelles***, 80 % of patients

---

[11] Ibid p 92.

who have undergone cognitive therapy experienced a significant and durable relief of their symptoms, including depression and anxiety.

Other diagnoses can include bloating (C.2), constipation (C.3) or functional diarrhoea (C.4), when IBS symptoms are present, but without any pain.

In the case of women, 40 percent of those diagnosed with IBS report having painful periods, and 50 percent have PMS[12].

According to Dr Georges Ghattas, it is generally useless to consult a specialist, since patients express more satisfaction when care is provided by a family physician than when it is provided by a specialist, especially when an organic diagnosis is excluded or unlikely.

D – Functional abdominal pain

The functional abdominal pain syndrome (D.1) is abdominal pain which lasts more than six months, is unrelated to intestinal functions and often necessitates a slowdown of activities. Patients with this syndrome tend to consult and have surgery more often than the population at large. Usually, doctors prescribe an antidepressant at a low dosage. A good doctor-patient relationship, regular consultations, a good stress and anxiety management program, and follow-up care to help fight depression are also recommended. A diagnosis of unspecified functional abdominal pain (D.2) is made whenever the pain is not found to be related to functional abdominal pain syndrome.

E – Functional disorder of the biliary tree and pancreas

Gall-bladder dysfunction (E.1) consists in biliary colic attacks when the gall-bladder has a normal appearance, i.e., when an ultra-sound of the abdomen does not reveal the presence of lithiasis (gallstones). More advanced tests may indicate microscopic gallstones. The effectiveness of a cholecystectomy is unpredictable and should be decided on an individual basis. Dysfunction of Oddi's sphincter

---

[12] Ibid p. 95.

(E.2) (a small valve located between the biliary tree and the intestine) may require specific treatments. However, mostly the problem is due to IBS or functional dyspepsia.

F – Functional abdominal pain

Functional fecal incontinence (F.1) consists of recurring involuntary defecation in the absence of a neurological or structural disorder of the intestinal wall. It affects approximately 30% of elderly people living in long-term facilities, but it is also found in almost a quarter of people suffering from diarrhoea-related IBS. In the case of constipated elderly people, the problem is usually treated by an osmotic laxative (lactulose), and when diarrhoea is predominant, with leporamide.

Anticholinergic medications[13] can be used to help prevent or relieve painful cramps and intestinal spasms (hyoscyamine sulphate, dicyclonine hydrochloride, clidinium, donnatal). These medications seem to also dry up secretions in the intestines and are generally not recommended for IBS patients.

Functional anorectal pain (F.2) can be divided into levator syndrome (F.2a), and *proctalgia fugax* (F.2b). In the absence of a structural or inflammatory disorder, the first type is characterized by rectal pain that lasts at least twenty minutes and may affect the patient for twelve weeks or more during the previous year. Muscle relaxants (methocarbamol, diazepam and cyclobenzeprine), anorectal massages and sits baths can be contemplated. *Proctalgia fugax* produces rare acute pain lasting from a few seconds to a few minutes; it subsequently disappears completely and is not felt in between defecation. In rare cases when this symptom occurs frequently, doctors may prescribe a salbutamol inhalation; others may suggest clonidine or amylnitrate.

Pelvic floor dyssynergia, or anism (F.3), extensively treated by Dr Devroede, consists of the contradictory contraction of the pelvic

---

[13]   Ibid, pp. 157-158.

floor, which occurs when a person bears down while defecating. Rather than relaxing the anal area, the patient contracts it to prevent defecation. The diagnosis requires a physiological investigation (anorectal manometry, electromyography of the external anal sphincter, balloon defecation test and defecography). Two thirds of the patients can learn, by means of biofeedback, to relax the pelvic floor during defecation.

Finally resent researches showed that IBS patients are prompt to proptosis, which is a contraction of back muscles and lowering down of diaphragm compressing organs and making the belly looking bigger. This is a physical impairment known to be specific and frequent in IBS cases. Causes and treatment are unknown.

For more information on the Rome criteria, consult: http://www.romecriteria.org . For Dr Poitras' articles (in French) consult: http://www.mauxdeventre.org .

Here are the tips found in the brochure *IBS and You*, quoted earlier:

1. If your doctor has made a definite diagnosis, stop worrying by asking yourself if it couldn't be "something else", such as the early stages of a cancer.
2. Avoid things which, in your experience, tend to aggravate your condition, such as triggering foods, people or thoughts (cognitive distortion).
3. Use medication to avoid attacks, for example, take an antidiarrheic before leaving the house when you fear that there will not be any bathrooms at your destination and you think you may have to go. Fight constipation by including fibre in your diet (provided that fibers do not have an irritating effect on you).
4. Try to find the sources of stress in your life and consider how you could reduce or manage them.
5. With professional help, try to determine what problems you are avoiding in your own life, and take the necessary measures to resolve them.

6. Learn to relax: you probably don't know how to go about it. Various strategies ranging from yoga to acupuncture to meditation can help, but remember that nothing is as effective as getting to know yourself (Did Socrates have IBS?).
7. Above all, decide who's in charge of your life – yourself or your intestine. Life is much easier when you decide that you are the one in charge (*easier said than done, especially when we feel guilty at letting our intestines decide for us*).

B) – THE MOST COMMON SYMPTOMS

• Gas and flatulence[14]

Abdominal bloating affects approximately two thirds of people suffering from IBS. In some people the pain lasts for days, with periods varying in intensity. In addition to evacuating the gas, another tactic is to reduce its production, which occurs during digestion, and avoid swallowing air as much as possible. According to pharmacist Patrick Viet-Quoc Nguyen, these abdominal symptoms can be divided into three categories:

1. eructation: noisy emission – through the mouth, either voluntary or not – of gas coming from the oesophagus, sometimes from the stomach;

---

[14] *Canadian Society of Intestinal Research*: http://www.badgut.com
Michael Oppenheim, M.D., *The Complete Book of Better Digestion – A Gut-Level Guide to Gastric Relief*, Rodale Press, Emmaus, Pennsylvania, 1990.
Perreault, Danielle. M. D. *Le Soleil*, Mars 28th 2004, p. A 15.
Viet-Quoc Nguyen, Patrick. Pharmacist, *Québec Pharmacie*, vol. 51, n° 7, July-August 2004, p. 572-576.
Jolicœur, Annie. Nutritionist, from *Du cœur au ventre*, AMGIF, vol. 2, n° 1, Spring 2002, p. 2-3.

2. meteorism: sensation of abdominal swelling attributed to the accumulation of gas in the stomach and intestines;
3. flatulence: gas accumulated in the intestines and expelled through the rectum.

Swallowed air

A study has shown that a normal individual produces from one to three litres of gas a day, 90% of which is made up of oxygen, nitrogen (NH_4) and CO_2, swallowed while eating or by reflex. The remainder, hydrogen and methane, is produced by the bacterial breakdown of food residues in the large intestine. We can swallow as much as a litre of air at every meal. Some people swallow twice as much air as water when they drink. Dr Oppenheim indicates that it is often difficult to make patients understand that their bloating is probably caused by the air they swallow.

Air that is swallowed remains in the stomach for some time before it is released through eructation or through a slow-paced transit in the small intestine, the large intestine, and finally the anus. A small quantity of it is absorbed by the aerobic bacteria and returned to the circulation (CO_2, H_2 and CH_4). Air stretches the stomach which may contain up to four and a half litres (a gallon and a half) of it. Gas may become painful, especially if it is associated with hiatal hernia, gastroesophageal reflux or gastric ulcer. A bloated stomach can exert pressure on the large intestine, occasionally creating cramps, contractions and spasms. The air accumulated in the large intestine is associated with constipation and diarrhoea. In general, the passage of air in the small intestine isn't painful. On average, a person passes gas (flatulence) in small quantities, approximately 12 times a day, and in the case of vegetarians, up to 25 times a day.

Most people who pass gas do not experience any discomfort. In the case of the inflammatory disease of the digestive system, or IDD, the passing of gas is slower (dysmotility) and more painful (hypersensitivity).

In the case of meteorism, patients apparently have a slower intestinal transit, or hypersensitivity to visceral stimuli, regardless of the quantity of gas.

It is in the morning that the digestive system holds the least amount of gas since there is no swallowing of air, or flatulence accumulating in the night. The amount of flatulence depends on the volume of air swallowed, on the nature and quantity of the air ingested, on meal frequency, the type of food, and on colon motility. The latter can be influenced by diet, medications, stress, and the volume of air already trapped in the digestive system. My recent experience showed me that there could be a fairly large amount of gas trapped in the digestive track even in the morning.

To reduce air intake you should avoid chewing gum, breathing while drinking, including liquids that are too hot, and wearing badly adjusted dental prostheses. You should not drink while eating. It is better to drink fifteen to thirty minutes prior to a meal, and from one to two hours following a meal. Blowing your nose, chronic pain and anxiety can also stimulate the swallowing reflex. Dr Michael Oppenheim tells his patients to keep their moths closed, including while eating, because some of them have the reflex of swallowing air... every time they breathe.

Bacteria

Another significant source of gas is the proliferation of bacteria. This can originate from a non-acidic stomach and caused by an insufficient production of gastric acid, from taking too many antacids, or from eating too much alkalinizing foods. When food stagnates in the small intestine of persons whose intestinal motor nerves have been damaged as in the case of some diabetics it can also produce gas.

Bacteria in the small intestine can produce large amount of gas. Bacteria in the large intestine could progress into the small intestine where food is less digested, so more prone to trigger gases. Some of the wastes produced by bacteria could pass through intestinal wall in the bloodstream. The immune system could respond by creating antibody complexes. The book IBS for Dummies[15] refers to a 2003 study that found that 84 percent of patients with IBS had abnormal breath test results suggesting small intestinal bacterial overgrowth. Antibiotic treatment improves outcome for many of these patients.

Other causes explain the presence of air in the oesophagus and stomach, including anxiety with hyperventilation, asthma, chronic obstructive pulmonary disease, hiatal hernia, gastric obstruction, reflux, abdominal wind, hypersalivation (chewing gum), pregnancy and smoking. In the case of meteorism and flatulence, we should add parasites, Crohn's disease, gall stones, diverticulitis, diabetes, hypothyroidism, food intolerance, as well as certain medications (anticholinergic or antidiarrheal agents).

Since the main cause of gas is the air we breathe, it seems fairly obvious that medications, herbal teas and other remedies available on the market to reduce their occurrence are generally ineffective. I tried simethicone (Ovol), and activated coal supplements, unsuccessfully. When we're full of gas, it is useful to evacuate it. For example, a Spanish study published in the *American Journal of Medicine* (referred to in *The Inside Tract* journal of January-February 2006) showed that eight normal adults to whom air has been injected in the small intestine released more air when they exercised than when they were idle. After two hours, they had released 90 percent of the air injected without exercise, but had released more air than had been injected when they exercised.

---

[15]   IBS for Dummies, p. 20-21.

- ### Gastroesophageal reflux (GERD) [16]

Regular heartburn (pyrosis), but also difficulty in swallowing, persistent cough, hoarseness and even asthma, are symptoms of gastroesophageal reflux disease (GERD). It occurs when the muscle ring separating the oesophagus and the stomach, the lower oesophageal sphincter, relaxes and allows gastric acid to rise. The mucus membrane of the oesophagus, more sensitive than the stomach membrane, produces a burning sensation when brought into contact with acid elements. One third of the population has had at least one episode of heartburn, while 10 percent experience them on a daily basis.

The mere act of lying down or belching after a meal can cause the food to rise up in the oesophagus (regurgitation). Violent exercise, such as exercises requiring that you bend down, heavy meals, eating fast or tight clothing have the same effect. If it occurs frequently, GERD causes an irritation or inflammation of the oesophagus (oesophagitis), or of the respiratory tract (frequent cough, hoarseness). If gastric juices are often in contact with the teeth, they may attack the tooth enamel.

A new study mentioned in the online magazine *E-santé* (www.e-sante.fr) confirms the relationship between GERD and weight, suggesting that weight loss helps limit acid reflux. These results stem from the well-known *Nurses' Health Study*, a survey of 10,000 nurses between the ages of 30 and 55 who were followed since 1976.

Oesophagitis is common among children and adults between the ages of 45 and 64. It can cause dysphagia (swallowing disorder) or bleeding (inflammation and ulcers). Persons who are obese or

---

[16] Mayo Clinic. *Les maladies de l'appareil digestif,* Lavoie & Broquet, p. 83-97.
Service Vie-Santé : http://www.servicevie.com/02Sante/Cle_des_maux/B/maux45.html
Online Magazine *E-santé* : http://www.e-sante.fr
Association des maladies gastro-intestinales fonctionnelles (AMGIF). *RGO - Le reflux gastro-œsophagien* : www.amgif.qc.ca

suffer from hiatal hernia, asthma, diabetes or peptic ulcers, as well as pregnant women, are liable to have this complaint. It seems that only medium to large-size hiatal hernias cause reflux. In the most severe cases, surgery can be considered.

After listening to your symptoms, your doctor may order an X-ray (to investigate possible ulcer), an endoscopy (to assess the risk of complications), a biopsy, a pHmetry (24-hour reflux) or an oesophageal manometry (pressure of the muscular function of the oesophagus and sphincter).

Stop smoking: tobacco is an emetic, a substance that makes you throw up by irritating the stomach and intestines. Eat smaller meals: large meal triggers unnecessary gut activity. "Stretching the stomach and the various sphincters sends messages of urgency down the entire intestinal tract.[17]" Cut down on fatty foods, especially ice cream (dairy products, fat and sugar at once) and strong alcoholic drinks lose excess weight and raise your headboard by 15 cm (6 inches), are helpful suggestions. Be aware that a lot processed low sugar foods have a higher content in fat to stay attractive. On the other hand, spicy foods are not involved in acid reflux. Proteins reinforce the sphincter of the lower oesophagus, provided these proteins are not combined with fatty foods. Straining (bearing down), especially while bending forward, should be avoided. Some medications should also be avoided, such as antispasmodics, calcium inhibitors, potassium and vitamin C tablets, non-steroid anti-inflammatory medications, sedatives and tranquilizers. Recommended medications include antacids, which however can cause diarrhoea and constipation; histaminic H2 receptor inhibitors which reduce acid secretion (Peptol, Tagamet, Pepcid, Axid, Zantac, etc.); proton pump inhibitors (Losec, Prevacid, Pantoloc) as well as prokinetics, which ease stomach emptying.

As I mentioned in my approach, eructation may also be used to expel gas that has accumulated in the stomach, and therefore reduce the pressure

---

[17]   Ibid, p. 316.

inside it. This method has allowed me to totally eliminate heartburns. However, when I neglect my evacuation exercises I feel irritation in my respiratory tract, my voice becomes hoarse (silent reflux) and, naturally, the heartburn returns if I don't pull myself together.

If you have heartburn more than twice a week, or if your symptoms are only temporarily relieved by antacids, you should see a doctor. The side effect of antacid is underdigestion in the stomach leading to meal for bacteria and yeast, than gas and diarrhoea. In severe cases that resist other treatments, surgery is an option.

• Asthma and gastroesophageal reflux

Gastric acid reflux in the oesophagus can trigger an asthma attack, so it is appropriate to treat gastroesophageal reflux in asthma patients. This is especially important in the case of children. Asthma is a chronic bronchial tube inflammation that can cause typical asthma attacks (difficult, wheezy breathing) and chronic cough.

The relationship between gastric acid reflux and asthma attacks has been known for a long time. When digestion starts the food is dissolved in the stomach by the action of gastric acid, which has hydrochloric acid as a component. The bolus does not attack the stomach, which is protected. In the rest of the digestive tract the acidity is mainly neutralized by the alkaline secretions of the small intestine. Physiologically, this acidic bolus should not rise into the oesophagus because it is prevented from doing so by a sphincter: the cardia.

When GERD is experienced, gastric acidity rises in the oesophagus. In addition to burning the walls of the oesophagus itself, acid reflux can go down into the bronchial tubes and cause local irritation, triggering asthma attacks. Yet, many asthma sufferers do not complain of reflux. A study shows that 62% of all asthmatics who do not present GERD symptoms have, in fact, a pathological pHmetry: they suffer from silent reflux. Their pHmetry was generally as disrupted as the one of patients with a clinical GERD and their asthma was as severe. Another study in which 128 asthmatic patients were surveyed revealed that almost half (53) suffered from GERD. Out of these 53, 48 had a wheezing cough – a classic sign of impending asthma attack – shortly after the reflux.

In practice, it is appropriate to identify and treat any GERD present in asthmatics. This is especially true in the case of infants and toddlers, for whom this is a still under diagnosed problem. In fact, children's cough is often caused by the many viral or bacterial infections they are likely to catch, and asthma is often overlooked. It should be considered at the slightest indication, especially if a chronic cough disturbs the child's sleep or is accompanied by wheezing. These are children in whom a possible GERD should be identified and treated as part of an asthma assessment.

In the case of asthma, whether or not a silent GERD is diagnosed, the technique for releasing stomach gas can probably help if, as in my case, the reflux stops within a few minutes after the air have been evacuated from the stomach.

• Constipation [18]

According to Dr Oppenheim, a good diet and regular exercise make constipation virtually impossible. Yet, according to certain estimates, constipation is a widespread complaint, affecting nearly 20% of people living in western countries. It is most reported by women, especially a week before period, and it tends to get worse as people

---

[18] Article of Réjean Dubé M. D., *Le Médecin du Québec*, vol. 37, n° 2, February 2002.
Article of Isabelle Hébert M. D., *E-santé* : http://www.e-sante.fr
Jacques Rogé, professor, *Le mal de ventre*, Éditions Odile Jacob, 1998.
Michael Oppenheim, M. D., *The Complete Book of Better Digestion: A Gut-Level Guide to Gastric Relief*, Rodale Press, Emmaus, Pennsylvania, 1990.
Article of Mickael Bouin, gastroenterologist « *La constipation fonctionnelle : un symptôme unique pour des mécanismes multiples* », *Du cœur au ventre*, AMGIF, Winter 2005, p. 2-3.
Article of Stéphane Lehman M. D., *E-santé* : http://www.e-sante.fr

get older. Most people who consult their doctor about this are not seriously ill. However, it is known that any damage on nerves or intestinal muscles due to IBS could trigger constipation.

According to Dr Mickael Bouin, for patients constipation means stools that are hard or difficult to expel. Doctors rely instead on a description based on the Rome criteria. To fit this description, the following two criteria must be present for at least twelve weeks, consecutive or not, during the previous year.

More than one time out of four, the patient must:
1. Make an effort to defecate;
2. Has hard or pellet like stools;
3. Has a sensation of incomplete evacuation;
4. Feels a blockage or an anal or rectal obstruction at the time of defecation;
5. Has to help himself/herself manually to defecate (manual evacuation).

Moreover, the norm is less than three defecations per week.

Functional constipation can be subdivided into four sub-groups: slow transit, pelvic floor dysfunction, irritable colon and the absence of a clear anomaly.

Slow transit

This type of constipation is characterized by the slower progress of the colon contents (colic inertia). It accounts for roughly a quarter of all constipation cases. Its source can be dietetic or cultural, or it can arise from a motor anomaly (decreased high magnitude peristaltic waves, or increased uncoordinated motor activity). This is where my assumption that constipation results from an accumulation of gas in the digestive system fits in: the large intestine feels like it is jammed up. Slow transit can be revealed by an X-ray. The patient swallows radio opaque markers and then radiological tests are administered to find out how fast these markers are progressing in the colon.

Pelvic floor dysfunction

Even when there is no transit abnormality, this dysfunction concerns rectal stool build-up that lasts for long periods (terminal constipation). It represents approximately half of all constipation cases. In pelvic floor dysfunction the external anal sphincter and pelvic floor muscles are not relaxed during defecation, when the person strains. There can also be anorectal dyschesia when defecation is incomplete or fecal matter remains in the rectum.

Defecation is a relatively complex process that involves reflexes as well as a voluntary activity. It happens that a patient bears down and retains the stools at the same time. This is called anism (also see the chapter concerning Dr Devroede's book).

According to Professor Rogé, this type of constipation is often seen in children who are forced to hold it in. Once the urge is inhibited it disappears, and over time this affects the perception of the initial urge. The child may develop chronic constipation (as in my case). For example, colopaths will give up the urge to relieve themselves in the morning, or they will force themselves to stay in the toilet for longer periods (bathroom reader). They may be tempted to bear down too hard during defecation and thus cause complications such as haemorrhoids or anal fissures.

Functional constipation

This diagnosis is made when the possibility of slow transit or IBS-related constipation have been waived aside. Slow transit represents approximately a quarter of all functional constipation cases.

Irritable bowel and anomaly

We refer to IBS-related constipation when abdominal pain is added to the clinical picture. When there is no anomaly, the constipated patient is often distressed.

Secondary causes of constipation

Constipation can result from the following: a congenital ailment, Hirschsprung's disease, obstruction, colon or rectal cancer, colic stenosis or anorectal diseases, anal fissure, proctitis, metabolic diseases (autoimmune hypercalcaemia, hyperparathyroidism, hypothyroidism, diabetes), celiac disease, neurological diseases, muscular medullary lesions, multiple sclerosis, visceral neuropathy or myopathy, Parkinson's, as well as certain medications (laxatives, anticholinergic drugs, narcotics, antiparkinsonian drugs, calcium inhibitor sedatives, antidepressants, convulsant antidote, diuretics, neuroleptic drugs, iron and calcium supplements).

Constipation and diet

According to Dr Isabelle Hébert, very restrictive weight loss diets are often accompanied by constipation. A lower calories and fibres intake may prevent an adequate intestinal transit. We know that fibres hydrate and increase the volume of fecal matter, which promotes the movement of the stool. Even if a diet is appropriate it will necessarily reduce fecal volume, which is often wrongly associated with constipation.

The food we eat must provide us with enough protein to maintain muscle health (1.3-1.4 g of protein per kg – or 0.01 once per pound – of body weight/day); enough vitamins and minerals (in the form of fruits and vegetables) to avoid nutritional deficiencies and enough fibre to facilitate intestinal transit. Finally, we should drink a litre and a half of water every day and exercise.

Constipation and ageing

Intestinal transit disorders are especially common in individuals who are over 65: more than one in two elderly people have this kind of complaint. Normal ageing impacts all bodily functions. Yet age doesn't slow down the intestinal transit. What decreases is overall muscle tone, especially perineal muscles, making defecation more difficult.

Generally, chronic diseases are the most significant risk factors in constipation. Ailments such as diabetes, thyroid dysfunction, kidney deficiency, Parkinson's, cerebral vascular diseases, depression, etc., can cause it. The risk increases when the diseases add up (diabetes and kidney failure; Parkinson's and depression, for instance).

When should you seek medical attention?

According to Dr Oppenheim, it is absolutely necessary to seek medical attention if you haven't defecated in ten days. However, you should see a doctor after only three days if you also experience abdominal pain, a fever, or vomiting.

Clinical assessment

When a patient consults for a recent problem, the doctor is on the lookout for a disease, especially if the patient is over fifty. Chronic constipation, however, suggests a functional origin. The doctor will question the patient about its appearance mode, its progress, medication, stool characteristics, diet, intestinal functioning schedule, etc. Recent constipation, a sudden change in the regularity or volume of the stools, especially in older people, are indications that more tests are needed to rule out organic lesions. The doctor will also check the family medical history (polyps and colon or rectal cancer).

The purpose of the clinical examination is to check for perineal prolapse, the anal reflex as well as the muscle tone of the sphincter at rest and during voluntary contraction.

The investigation

Blood tests can reveal a treatable disease (hypothyroidism) or give a preliminary assessment of colon cancer. An X-ray and an endoscopy are generally administered to new patients over fifty years old, or when a new symptom has surfaced. Often, a sedative medication is given or drugs that induce amnesia so that you are relaxed for the procedure and don't remember anything afterward. I passed an endoscopy in 2010, and in fact I don't remember what happened, out of the doctor waking me up to show me the light through the lower right of my belly skin. If the constipation fails to respond to suitable hydration, higher fibre content and a simple laxative, this suggests a refractory constipation. A specialized assessment can then be contemplated. The doctor could order more tests (transit measurement, anorectal manometry and defecography), or refer the patient to a specialist.

Practical tips

Get moving: a sedentary lifestyle and confinement in bed reduces motility. Whenever possible, a daily walk is recommended.

Eat well: loss of appetite and a decrease in the dietary fibre intake fosters constipation. Eat fruits and vegetables regularly.

Never let the urge pass: we should go to the bathroom when we feel we need to. We can also go at fixed times. Microenemas can also be used to maintain regularity.

Drink sufficiently: a glass of water in the morning can trigger the urge, but drinking frequently during the day is not always effective in preventing constipation. Since the drinking reflex wanes as we get older, we must force ourselves to drink one litre to a litre and a half a day.

Help yourself: provided you follow your doctor's recommendations, taking laxatives, even daily, is acceptable. However, stay away from the latest miracle treatments sold over the counter. Self-medication, even for constipation, should be avoided.

Medical treatment

Doctors are likely to suggest an increase in fibre intake, but according to Dr Oppenheim there is such a thing as eating too much fibre. He mentions a patient who needed emergency surgery when a mass of dietary fibre obstructed his intestines. A simple way to measure adequate fibre intake is to watch the stools as you flush. If fecal matter continues to float on the surface without flushing you are probably consuming too many fibres. Fibres can also cause flatulence, something we should get used to. Since fibres are highly water absorbent, Dr Oppenheim recommends drinking two glasses of liquid with every meal, and adding a glass of water for each additional teaspoon of fibre (bran or psyllium). However, you should take care not to drink too much. A simple rule to follow is to check the colour of urine. If the urine is translucent, you should reduce your liquid intake until its colour turns yellowish. You should also remain active and eat a good breakfast since these two factors stimulate digestive functions.

A saline laxative such as milk of magnesia can be considered. We can also try a fecal emollient (sodium docusate). Also available are hyperosmotic agents (lactulose, polyethyleneglycol, and sorbitol). Your doctor will probably avoid stimulating laxatives such as sennodides or bisacodyl. The use of glycerine suppositories or enemas is generally limited. It seems that no prokinetic agent on the market has an effect on colonic function.

According to Dr Bouin, most over-the-counter medication is effective (Colace, Senokot, Dulcolax, and Solflax). He favours stimulating laxatives when colonic transit is slow. However, these laxatives seem to be too painful for IBS-related constipation. The International Foundation for Functional Gastrointestinal Disorders found that 79 percent of people with IBS take over-the-counter laxatives[19].

Mineral oil[20] is the most common lubricant to help the stool to move through the intestine. The side effects include malabsorption of vitamins A, D, E, and K creating at term vitamin deficiency symptoms.

Biofeedback can be prescribed, but it seems to be more effective in cases of anism. The patient's and the therapist's motivation, the frequency and intensity of the rehabilitation program, as well as the support of a psychologist tend to improve success.

---

[19]   IBS for Dummies, p. 152.
[20]   Ibid. p. 154.

Surgical treatment

When constipation persists despite intensive medical treatment, the surgeon may consider a total colonectomy with ileorectal anastomosis. This surgery will solve the evacuation problem but not the abdominal pain and bloating.

- ## Diarrhoea [21]

The main causes of diarrhoea are viruses (60 to 80% of cases) and bacteria found in water and food (especially meat, seafood, eggs, cheese, and mayonnaise). When you eat in fast-food restaurants, at buffets or food stands, the food may be contaminated because of the way it is handled and reheated without the bacteria being destroyed. Child-care centres, hospitals and chronic care facilities are most vulnerable to this type of contamination.

Diarrhoea occurs while too much liquid is produce in the intestine. So drinking too much liquid could trigger diarrhoea. But the most widely known cause is IBS itself.

Gastric surgery reduces gastric acid – a protection against bacteria – other causes also include antibiotics and magnesium antacids. Generally, the symptoms are more important on the first day, and last from three to seven days.

Chronic diarrhoea is often caused by intestinal or colonic inflammation, food intolerance or parasites. Gallbladder surgery can also cause bile leak. The cause can also be psychological. Finally, it is widespread among people suffering from IBS.

---

[21] Michel Tulin, M. D. gastroenterologist, *Hôpital du Haut-Richelieu*, Saint-Jean-sur-Richelieu; http://www.e-sante.fr
Catherine Feldman, M. D. : http://www.e-sante.fr
Christine Collard, *Quotipharm* : http://www.quotipharm.com
IBS for Dummies, p. 70.

For the authors of IBS for Dummies, acute episodes of infectious diarrhoea, like dysentery, can scrape off layers of cells from the delicate mucus lining of the gut. That lining contains enzymes that digest wheat, dairy, and fruit. Lacks of these enzymes can provoke lactose or gluten intolerance. While these nutrients are not well digested, they ended up in the large intestine where fermentation and putrefaction feed bacteria and yeast that are gas-forming organisms.

As indicated by Dr Oppenheim, the closer to the anus the disorder causing the diarrhoea occurs, the quicker you should respond to the urgent need.

When should you see your doctor?

- You've had diarrhoea for over a week;
- You've lost weight;
- Your diarrhoea is accompanied by fever, bloody stools or strong abdominal cramps;
- You notice the presence of mucus (transparent liquid) or pus (a thick foul-smelling yellow or green discharge) in your stools;
- Your mouth, lips and tongue are abnormally dry;
- You notice a decrease in urine volume;
- You are pregnant and experience one or more of these symptoms.

Medical examination

Patients are generally given a complete examination and the doctor may order a stool culture. The Comprehensive Digestive Stool Analysis (CDSA) is a panel of tests that looks for evidence of maldigestion, malabsorption, and abnormal intestinal bacteria end ecology. Also a simple stool test collected at home could be sent to a specialty lab that conducts the CDSA to count also the amount of organisms present and can tell you if you have too much or even to little of a particular bacteria or yeast. One of such a lab can be reach on its web site www.gsdl.com [22]. Depending on the seriousness of the problem, blood tests may be ordered or more rarely, a rectoscopy, X-rays and an intestinal biopsy in the case of chronic diarrhoea. In blood tests, a complete blood count will rule out celiac disease (low hemoglobin counts), protein deficiency or zinc deficiency (low white cells counts), a chem screen will rule out liver and kidney problems, and CA-125 test, will rule out ovarian cancer[23].

The biological balance sheet distinguishes between acute diarrhoea related to a digestive infection from chronic diarrhoea (intestinal malabsorption).

According to the nature of the anomaly investigated, the following tests can be ordered:

- For cases of diarrheic malabsorption, the d-xylose absorption test using a simple sugar mostly absorbed in the jejunum, could be administered. This test indicates the absorption capacity of the intestinal surface involved, and helps diagnose celiac disease or steatorrhea. The Schilling test (absorption of the B12 vitamin) also reveals intestinal malabsorption and helps diagnose Biermer's disease;
- A stool culture can underscore the infectious origin of the diarrhoea (*Escherichia coli*, salmonella, shigella, campylobacter, etc.). It is performed when the patient has a fever or when the stools are bloody or slimy;
- A parasitological examination of the stools is done when the diarrhoea is accompanied by nausea, vomiting or abdominal pain occurring particularly when returning from a trip.

---

[22] Ibid, p. 328.
[23] Ibid, p. 323.

The usual treatment[24]

An antibiotic, an antidiarrheal agent or proper hydration usually does the trick. If the dehydration is severe and accompanied by fever and bloody stools, the patient is hospitalized to be rehydrated intravenously. Lomotil that slows down intestinal movements could be prescribed for a short period of time since, as an opiate drug, it is addictive. Imodium also slows down intestinal movements and it enhances the resting internal anal sphincter tone. It is not addictive, but it does not have any effect on abdominal pain or distension. For this reason, it is not recommended for IBS patients. Questran, a bile acid binding agent is also used for treatment of cholesterol. Abdominal pain, bloating, constipation, gas, a feeling of fullness and nausea are its side effects.

In the case of antibiotics, if you had to take high doses of IV antibiotics, that could leave room for Clostridium difficile which is resistant to most antibiotics. Normally, if you have to take antibiotics, make sure you take probiotic supplements or eat organic, plain yogurt that contains Lactobacillus acidophilus and/or Bifidobacteria to build up your good bacteria.[25]

Lactose intolerance

If lactose intolerance is what causes the chronic diarrhoea, eliminating the culprit, or taking Lactaid, should be sufficient. Dairy products can be reintroduced progressively in small amounts. With young children milk can be replaced with a soy-based formula. You must preferably use soy products made with fermented soy which are easier to digest.

The diagnostic test[26] for lactose intolerance is called hydrogen breath test. First, you will breathe into a machine to obtain a baseline level of hydrogen (parts per million). Then, you will drink a lactose sugar

---

[24]   Ibid, pp. 149-150.
[25]   Ibid, p. 294.
[26]   Ibid, p. 137.

liquid dissolved in water, and you will breathe into a machine every 30 minutes for up to 3 hours. A rise of greater than 20 parts of hydrogen per million within the 3 hours is diagnostic of lactose intolerance.

Traveller's diarrhoea

According to Dr Catherine Feldman, traveller's diarrhoea is most often caused by an infection, generally a bacteria (especially *Escherichia coli*), sometimes a parasite (an amoeba, for example), and rarely a virus. It is one of the elements that set off traveller's diarrhoea from the viral diarrhoea common in Western Europe.

Germs are most often transmitted through contaminated foods that are prepared well in advance of a meal, and sometimes stored under dubious conditions. Prevention is difficult, however, because it is based on food hygiene rules that are difficult to apply.

Many travellers, before leaving on a trip, ask their doctor for antibiotics to prevent travellers' trots. Antibiotics are not prescribed right away because they entail side-effects and can build bacterial resistance. The people most at risk are the ones who need them, that is, insulin-dependent diabetics, AIDS patients, people with high blood pressure who take diuretics, or those who carry chronic intestinal inflammatory diseases such as Crohn's disease or ulcerous colitis.

Practical tips

Drink a lot to avoid dehydration (this is very important in the case of young children and elderly people): water, juice, degasified 7-Up, or a commercial electrolyte preparation (mineral salts). Sweet beverages for sportsmen and women supply electrolytes and sugar (which helps the intestines absorb liquids) could be taken. Or you can mix boiled water (1 L or 1 pint) with a pinch of salt and bicarbonate, 30 ml (2 Tbsp.) of sugar and 120 ml (1/2 cup) of apple juice.

Eat lightly, a little of everything, except dairy products and fibres. However, if you have strong abdominal cramps or if you vomit, it is better for you to fast, have something to drink and get some rest.

When you rest in bed the intestines have more time to do their work. When you feel better, start eating progressively again, choosing digestible foods: light soups, ripe bananas, toast. Better for you will be to eat six light meals a day than three big ones. Stay away from milk, coffee, tea, alcohol, coke or tap water, which tend to stimulate the intestines. Avoid foods high in carbohydrates such as bran and pasta, as well as cabbage and vegetables. If you eat simple carbs, especially refined sugar, with protein or fat, the sugar from the carbs gets trapped in your stomach where fermentation will produce gas.

If you think that the cause of your diarrhoea is some food you've eaten and that you are running a fever, do not take an antidiarrheic medication such as Imodium without consulting your doctor. It could slow down the elimination of the bacteria.

To avoid heartburn-related diarrhoea, choose an antacid that contains aluminum hydroxy rather than a magnesium-based antacid.

Wash your hands carefully when preparing a meal. Parasitic infections are also transmitted by hands. You should use your own soap and towels.

You could also try probiotic supplements or foods that contain beneficial bacteria such as *lactobacillus*, which are identical to the bacteria naturally present in intestinal flora. Their role is to prevent the proliferation of harmful bacteria. Some yeasts (*saccharomyces boulardii*) are known to prevent post-antibiotic diarrhoea and colitis. Many preparations are also said to restore intestinal flora (Bacilor, *Lyo-Bifidus*). However, it seems that pasteurization deactivates these bacteria in foods.

Medication

Most authors consider that taking medication to alleviate diarrhoea is not necessarily helpful, and that it is better to consult a health care professional first. Some patients should even avoid over-the-counter medications.

Intraluminal adsorbing agents: Attapulgite (Actapulgite), which is not available in some countries or other clays (diosmectite of Smecta) reduce the number of stools and the duration of a diarrheic episode. They do not reduce hydroelectrolitic loss so it is considered a back-up treatment.

Antibiotics: widely used in cases of acute diarrhoea caused by invasive bacterial infections, or chronic diarrhoea resulting from inoperable intestinal anomalies (blind loop syndrome, diverticulosis of the small intestine, etc.). Cholera, typhoid, shigellosis, severe cases of salmonella, typhoid fever, require this treatment. Tetracyclins are used to treat acute secretory forms, and lactamins, the bloody forms. Other types of antibiotics are used to treat specific problems.

Antisecretory medications: racecadotril (Tiorfan) is used to treat adult acute diarrhoea but it is not available in some countries.

Intestinal antiseptics: treat amoebiasis (potentially toxic for the optic nerve) as well as acute bacterial episodes without an invasive disease.

Transit: opiates slow down the transit and regulate water and electrolyte exchanges. They are used in cases of severe diarrhoea (Arestal, Imodium, Imossel, etc.). Atropine is sometimes combined with a transit moderator such as diphenoxylate (Diarsed) so as to exercise an antispasmodic activity and reduce pain.

In my case, large amount of gases in the digestive track is sometimes a trigger for diarrhoea. It seems that they distort the normal function of the large intestine enough to provoke diarrhoea. Getting rid of them reduces pain, diarrhoea, and improves regularity.

• Gastroenteritis [27]

According to Dr Isabelle Hébert, gastroenteritis is not the same as a bilious attack. It is rather a highly infectious ailment that often affects school children or family members, especially during winter. Symptoms of gastroenteritis include acute diarrhoea and abdominal cramps sometimes accompanied by nausea, vomiting, fever, aches and pains.

Viral gastroenteritis: unwashed hands

Germs are transported by fecal matter and are transmissible by the hands, when touching a doorknob or an object handled by other people, like money or food. In general, children do not wash their hands thoroughly (using hot water and for at least fifteen seconds) before they eat.

Bacterial gastroenteritis: food

Salmonella, less frequent but more severe, is the most common culprit found in the food we eat (meat, eggs, dairies). Colon bacilli found in meat and milk are also responsible.

Viral gastroenteritis is cured within a few days. As mentioned earlier, antispasmodic and antidiarrheic medications can alleviate the pain. An anti-residue diet (fibre free) is recommended: no raw fruits or vegetables, no milk or starchy foods except rice. You have to drink lots of liquids and feel free to seek relief. If your symptoms persist (fever) see your doctor. Blood tests and a stool culture reveal the presence of the guilty agent. Antibiotics, antispasmodic drugs or probiotics (*lactobacillus casei, lactobacillus acidophilus*) may be prescribed. Their purpose is to rebuild intestinal flora. It has the ability to break down sugar into lactic acid which in turn kills yeast.

---

[27]   Isabelle Hébert, M. D., *E-santé* : http://www.e-sante.fr
      Article of Mickael Bouin, Gastroentorologist, « *Le syndrome de l'intestin irritable : les pistes de recherche* », *Du cœur au ventre*, AMGIF, Winter 2006, p. 2-3.

To prevent viral gastroenteritis, wash your hands thoroughly after going to the bathroom, before cooking a meal or sitting down at table, or before a snack. Thoroughly clean the kitchen utensils that come into contact with raw meat, fish or eggs before using them again. It is recommended to always wash fruits and vegetables. When you have an infection, get much rest, and do not kiss anyone!

According to the 1999 Gwee study conducted with 94 patients who had suffered from infectious bacterial gastroenteritis, 23% presented an IBS a year after they were first surveyed, while they had none previously. The longer the infection lasts the greater the risk of developing IBS. It is estimated that from five to fifteen percent of all IBS cases are people who suffer from infectious IBS. We know that from five to twenty percent of bacterial gastroenteritis will develop into IBS within six months to a year after the infection. However, half of the cases are cured from IBS after six years of development.

- **Migraine** [28]

It seems that less than half of all migraine sufferers have been diagnosed as such, which means that only one-third of them get treatment. A simple test comprising three questions was developed recently: Migraine ID. The criteria developed by the *International Headache Society* were used to draw up a first questionnaire that was tested on 450 patients. Subsequently, these patients had a

---

[28] Isabelle Eustache, M. D., *E-santé* : http://www.e-sante.fr
Article of Pierre-René de Cotret and Marie-Michèle Mantha, M. Sc., *Passeportsanté.net* :
http://www.passeportsante.net/fr/Maux/Problemes/Fiche.aspx?doc=insomnie_pm
Article of Stéphane Ledoux M. D., « *La migraine : ce qu'il faut garder en tête* », *Le Clinicien*, May 2004, p. 67-72. : http://www.stacommunications.com/journals/leclinicien/2004/May/PDF/067.pdf

consultation with a specialist. The comparison helped eliminate questions that were not specific enough, until three questions left:

1. Have your activities been restricted by headaches for a day or more during the past three months?
2. Do you experience nausea or stomach pain when you have headaches?
3. Are you bothered by light when you have headaches?

Two positive answers out of three provide an 81% sensitivity level and a predictive value of 93%. It seems that this mini-test is sufficient to establish a pre-diagnosis. The mini-test could also encourage patients to consult so that they may receive the most appropriate treatment for their particular case.

Naturally, this test cannot replace a consultation with a specialist. It is interesting to note that a test with such a predictive value includes a question on nausea and stomach pain. According to Dr Stéphane Ledoux, the clinician must first make a reliable diagnosis. There are international criteria for every primary (without any structural lesion) and secondary headaches. The criteria for migraines without auras – the most common – are:

At least five previous attacks, including:

1. Attacks lasting from 2 to 72 hours (when there is no treatment);
2. Attacks that include at least two of these characteristics (unilateralism, pulsatility, moderate to severe pain intensity, aggravated by routine physical activities);
3. Attacks that are accompanied by at least an occurrence of nausea or vomiting, photophobia or phonophobia;
4. Clinical examination between attacks turns out normal.

The presence of an aura is not crucial in making this diagnosis since auras are only involved in 31% of the cases. Clinicians must distinguish between this type of migraine and that caused by an episodic tension headache, which requires a different kind of care.

Migraines are a global sensory hypersensitivity phenomenon (sensitivity to noise, light, smells and head movements). This hypersensitivity is not found in tension headaches.

Nowadays, migraine is considered to be an episodic dysfunction of some cerebral regions. It is therefore a chronic disease. However, it can generally be controlled by using a pharmacological approach.

Migraines are distinguishable from regular headaches by their duration and intensity, and the presence of other symptoms. The pain is often perceived as a shooting or pulsating pain inside the cranium. Migraines interfere with vision and cause nausea, vomiting and cold sweats. They can be preceded by an aura (auras are visual effects taking the form of lightning flashes, brightly coloured lines or temporary vision loss). Migraines occur at a rate varying from a few days a year to three to four times a month. They are rarely a daily occurrence. Some 10 to 20% of the population are believed to suffer from this disease.

The mechanics of a migraine

Little is known about how migraines work. The consensus is that they are caused by a swelling and inflammation of the blood vessels enveloping the brain.

Warning signs of upcoming migraines include difficulty in expressing oneself, excessive yawning, neck stiffness, irritability and increased sensitivity to noise, light and smells.

People whose parents currently suffer or have been suffering from migraines are at higher risk of being affected by the disease. In the case of women, hormonal changes are believed to have a triggering effect on migraines, since two-thirds of all women who get them do so during their period. For women suffering from IBS in that case, 50 % perceived an increase in gas production and pain in digestive track. The migraine attacks generally begin at puberty and often disappear when a woman is in her fifties.

Several factors are known to trigger a migraine attack; they vary from one person to the next. Everyone should learn to recognize these triggering factors. The main factors are stress, hunger, a change in health habits, changes in atmospheric pressure, bright lights or strong noises, too much or too little exercise, perfume, cigarette smoke, unusual smells. Some medications, including analgesics, oral contraceptives and hormone replacement therapy can also be the source of migraine.

Approximately 15 to 20% of all people suffering from migraines mention that some foods trigger their attacks. The foods most often incriminated are alcohol, chocolate, yogurt, fermented or marinated foods, monosodium glutamate, aspartame, caffeine or the lack of caffeine.

Prevention

To identify the triggering elements of an attack it is recommended to keep a diary in order to keep tabs on the food eaten in the last 24 hours, on the symptoms, on one's psychological condition and on external conditions (bright lights, noises, etc.). Precursory symptoms should also be recorded since their presence can facilitate treatment.

Unconventional approaches

Biofeedback and autogenous training can sometimes be more effective in preventing migraine than medication. The effect of relaxation is acknowledged by the Canadian Medical Association. A hypoallergenic diet without cow's milk, wheat, eggs and oranges has proven effective in a number of cases.

Phytotherapy and supplements

Health Canada authorizes allegations about the connection between feverfew and the prevention of migraine. Petasite has also been shown to be useful but there is little scientific data to support these claims.

A number of studies have confirmed the usefulness of magnesium (trimagnesium dicitrate) in significantly reducing the frequency and intensity of migraine attacks. Chronic magnesium deficiency[29] affects about 80 percent of the North American population. It is even more common in people with constipation. Moreover, calcium cannot function without magnesium. If you have been told that you have a potassium deficiency, you likely have a magnesium deficiency as well. If there is too much calcium and not enough magnesium, you can get muscle spasms or cramps, tics, nerve tingling, nerve pain, premature labour, or preeclampsia of pregnancy. The book IBS for Dummies recommend magnesium citrate like Mag Max-O and Narural Calm which you can take in small amount. If it creates diarrhoea, you can use magnesium glycinate or magnesium taurate which not seem to have laxative effect.

Medical treatments

Typically, migraine sufferers will turn to self-medication without obtaining any specific or sustainable relief, and with the added risk of having drug-induced headaches. It is probably best to see your doctor.

All treatments, whatever they may be, seem to be more effective when they are administered as soon as the precursory signs appear. Thus, taking aspirin, ibuprofen (Advil, Motrin, etc.) or non-steroid anti-inflammatory drugs can often stop a mild migraine attack in its tracks. If not, your doctor may suggest triptans (rizatriptan, naratriptan, and zolmitriptan). These drugs mimic the action of serotonin, which causes blood vessels to contract. Ergotamine (Ergomar, Cafergot) can also be prescribed as a pain reliever.

The purpose of prophylactics is to prevent an attack. They are prescribed only to people who suffer from frequent migraines. The most common medications used are beta blockers and calcium inhibitors (they help improve blood flow), low doses of tricyclic antidepressants and B2 vitamin.

---

[29] IBS for Dummies, pp. 170-171.

Any overuse of symptomatic treatment (including triptans) tends to increase the frequency of headaches. These treatments can lead to daily chronic headaches related to an overconsumption of medications.

Practical tips

When an attack occurs what we should do is lie down in a dark, quiet room, apply a cold compress on the forehead, massage the scalp and apply pressure on the temples.

In my case I need around two hours of evacuation exercises to get rid of a migraine. Afterwards I am left with a slight headache but I can remain active and exercise. Moreover, the exercise allows me to get a better quality of sleep, which means that the next day after a migraine my headache is usually gone. Although this book does not especially deal with migraines, to me it is obvious that it could form the basis of another book on this subject since the exercises described here seem not to have been discussed elsewhere.

- **Vagal faintness** [30]

Faintness, or syncope, is a loss of consciousness caused by a drop of the blood flow, and consequently of the brain's oxygen supply. The vagal condition is the most frequent cause of this ailment. We refer to it as "vagal" because it relates to the excessive stimulation of the pneumogastric nerves that control internal organs such as the lungs, the blood vessels, the heart and the stomach. This condition often stems from cardiocirculatory arrest, or a heartbeat disorder. It is accompanied by muscle relaxation and pallor of the face. It is often preceded by a sensation of heat, weakness, sweating or blurred vision. Several factors are at play in this kind of faintness attack: strong emotions, acute pain, heat, standing up for long periods,

---

[30] *Guide familial des symptômes*, Sante et Fides Edition, in Famili-Prix Inc. : http://www.famili-prix.com
Philippe Presles, M. D., *E-santé* : http://www.e-sante.f

stress, fatigue or alcohol consumption. Unfortunately, there is no treatment for vagal faintness at this time.

As opposed to faintness related to heart disease, there is no cardiac risk involved in vagal faintness. According to an American longitudinal study (*Framingham*) conducted with 8,000 participants concerning the causes of faintness, in 36.6% of cases the cause was unknown, the vagal condition explained 21.2% of the cases, cardiac disorders 9.5%, and orthostatic causes related to low blood pressure, 9.4%. In subjects who suffered a cardiac syncope, the risk of dying increased twofold; the risk of suffering a heart attack or dying from a coronary was increased by 2.7; and the risk of a cerebrovascular accident, by 2.

Practical tips

Patients should lie down and remain in this position until they feel better. When a person has regular attacks it is best to avoid standing in the same position for a long time, avoid heat, dehydration and alcohol.

If you see someone fainting, place him on his back and raise his legs. You can also apply a cold damp towel on their forehead.

A situation like this is considered an emergency if the person doesn't wake up within the next two or three minutes, has convulsions, loses consciousness repeatedly, has chest pains, is paralysed on one side of the body, or has an intense headache.

When I suffered from acute indigestion I used to faint. That was happening almost one time each year. But this is not happening anymore. However, it could come back if I stop doing my exercises.

• Hemerrhoids [31]

Hemorrhoids are similar to varicose veins (abnormal dilation, sometimes permanent, of the veins located around the anus). In adults, the onset of hemorrhoids is quite frequent. According to Dr Oppenheim, it is the price to pay for standing upright. Constipation and advanced pregnancy contribute to their development. They can be located in the upper part of the rectum (internal hemorrhoids) or around the anus (external hemorrhoids). They can cause acute pain and even bleeding.

According to Pr Rogé, over 70% of subjects suffering from IBS present or previously presented anorectal manifestations, such as emission of blood through the anus, hemorrhoids, anal fissures or anal itching. In the case of bloody stools, you absolutely must consult your doctor. A rectal exam to find whether you have hemorrhoids is not so frightening. Just remember that a doctor's finger is much narrower than the stool that passes through the anus. The itching can be caused by a number of things: extruding hemorrhoids, old fissures, *candida albicans*, infections, germs (streptococcus), or simply the regular presence of soft stools. Itching can be self-maintained by scratching. We have to make sure that the perianal region is clean, even going so far as wiping ourselves after passing gas that is especially humid. However, generally we should not wipe ourselves too much because it can cause skin irritation. A neutral soap (less irritating) can be used to maintain the perianal region perfectly clean. This will prevent dermatitis of the anal folds, which is the primary cause of non-stop itching.

---

[31] Isabelle Eustache, M. D., *E-santé*, Novembre 27th 2000. : http://www.e-sante.fr
Article of Philippe Presles M. D., *E-santé*, Octobre 13th 2004 :
http://www.e-sante.fr/magazine/article.asp?idArticle=7955&idRubrique =214&urldesc= A4H%c3%a9morro%c3%afdesefficacit%c3%a9confirm %c3%a9d
Jacques Rogé, professor, *Le mal de ventre*, Éditions Odile Jacob, Paris, 1998; http://www.odilejacob.fr

Very sharp pain

When it is violent and unbearable, the pain is usually caused by the constriction of a vein forming an outgrowth outside the anus. The formation of blood clots inside the vein can also cause sharp pain (hemorrhoidal thrombosis) with swelling of the vein, which becomes bluish and hard to the touch.

Harmless but troublesome bleeding

The bleeding, or hemorrhoidal rectorragy, is caused by lesions of the small blood vessels irrigating the anus. It is triggered by passing stools, is bright red and generally harmless.

A proctological exam is crucial

A proctological exam includes a rectal examination, an examination of the edge of the anus, and an anuscopy (examination of the anus using a tube equipped with an optical system). It is not enough to prescribe medication or ask for it. An anuscopy is essential because any anal anomaly (bleeding, pain, irritation, and lumps) can be the sign of a serious disease, including very serious ones such as colorectal cancer. The examination helps specify a diagnosis and rapidly sets the appropriate care in motion, to avoid aggravating the condition and increase the chances of a cure.

When should you seek treatment?

Hemorrhoids should be treated as soon as they cause significant discomfort, associated with pain and heavy bleeding. Your doctor has to make sure that this condition doesn't mask underlying ailments such as venereal disease or cancer. If a treatment turns out to be necessary, it should be remembered that there are medications for this disease but that they are only moderately effective. As for ambulatory treatments (minor surgeries, shots, ligatures), their use is limited. Surgery is the only intervention that can cure hemorrhoids permanently, but it is a solution that should be contemplated only if hemorrhoids cause serious health problems.

Medicinal treatment

The medicinal treatment for hemorrhoids generally combines several types of substances: laxatives to fight constipation, anti-inflammatory medications, and medications designed to improve circulation and venous tonicity. However, American experts have shown that only Daflon, a flavonoid-based medication, is effective. It heightens the resistance of small blood vessels and venous tone, which in turn reduces the bleeding caused by hemorrhoids.

In my case, as you know, I solved this problem by doing the anal contraction exercises.

• Insomnia [32]

Insomnia is characterized by a set of sleeping disorders that give one the impression of not getting enough sleep, or a good quality of sleep, or sleep that is not refreshing. We can generally identify three main types of insomnia, which are classified according to degree: acute insomnia, which lasts less than two weeks, subacute insomnia, which lasts between two weeks and six months, and chronic insomnia, which persists for more than six months. We can distinguish occasional and transitory insomnia, whose causes are easily discernible, from chronic insomnia. A person can have difficulty

---

[32] Article of Robert Dehin, Jocelyne Aubry and Marie-Michèle Mantha, M. Sc., *Passeportsanté.net* :
http://www.passeportsante.net/fr/Maux/Problemes/Fiche.aspx?doc=insomnie_pm
Article of Charles Ducroux, *Le Quotidien du pharmacien*, Septembre 2006 : http://www.quotipharm.com/journal/index.cfm?dnews=122998&newsId=23&fuseaction=viewarticle&DArtIdx=376351
Statistique Canada, Tjepkema M, Insomnie – Rapports sur la santé, vol. 17, n° 1, Novembre 2005, http://www.statcan.ca/Daily/Francais/051116/q051116a.htm
Article of Adrienne Gaudet, M. D., Pierre Savard, M. D., and Pascale Brillon, Ph. D., *Le Clinicien*, Octobre 2002, pp 75-84 :
http://www.stacommunications.com/journals/leclinicien/images/pdfoctclinicien/insomia.pdf

falling asleep, wake up during the night or wake up prematurely. In addition to the fatigue, the somnolence, the irritability and the poor concentration, insomnia is also known to aggravate digestive problems, migraines and muscle pain.

Among the causes we naturally find the gastroduodenal ulcer and gastroesophageal reflux, as well as a number of stimulating medications such as cortisone, beta blockers and antidepressants. All forms of stress can stimulate the waking system: excessive noise, chronic anxiety, intellectual or physical hyperactivity. Worries, relational difficulties, depression, manic state, phobias are also potential causes of insomnia. It seems that women with IBS are more susceptible to stress. They have higher level of stress hormones and chemicals than women who do not have IBS[33].

What are the diagnostic criteria?

Your doctor will consider that you suffer from insomnia if the time it takes you to fall asleep, or the time you spend being awake after first falling asleep exceeds thirty minutes, if your total sleeping period is under six and a half hours, or if the time you spend asleep is less than 85% of the time spent lying in bed. These problems must occur three nights or more in a week and last more than a month. The insomnia must cause psychological distress or difficulty with the social, family or occupational functioning.

According to Statistics Canada, one out of seven Canadians aged 15 or older experienced insomnia on a regular basis. Insomniacs sleep an average of six and a half hours a night, which is one hour less than subjects who get adequate sleep. Finally, almost one third of insomniacs take medications for their problem.

---

[33] IBS for Dummies, p. 101.

Phytotherapy

Phytotherapy is especially rich in various forms of sedative remedies. Linden and lemon balm are known for their relaxing properties. Lemon balm is used to treat mild nervous symptoms including restlessness and insomnia. Valerian roots, as well as the German Camomile, are effective in treating restlessness and sleeping disorders caused by nervousness. They are recognized by the World Health Organization.

In the case of acute or subacute insomnia, the treatment by the so-called "stimulus control" of behaviours is considered effective. It consists of scrupulously following a few directions for at least a month: getting up at set times, using the bedroom only for sleep or sexual activity, not remaining in bed while awake for more than twenty or thirty minutes (instead try to get up, engage in a relaxing activity and go back to bed when you get sleepy), avoiding naps.

Medication

If insomnia persists, a consultation is needed. Sleeping pills, generally benzodiazepins, may be prescribed. They are not for long-term use because they can lead to addiction, tolerance and withdrawal symptoms, including digestive problems. A new hypnotic drug like zopiclone, which doesn't seem to induce tolerance, addiction or memory problems, is recommended for the treatment of transitory and short-term insomnia.

Chronic insomnia requires a specific treatment. In the case of anxiety, depression or psychological disorders, your doctor may prescribe antidepressants to relieve the insomnia. He could also refer you to a psychologist or psychiatrist. When the insomnia is caused by pain, analgesics are an option.

Practical tips

It is also recommended to maintain a healthy lifestyle: avoid all stimulants (coffee, tea, vitamin C, Coca-Cola), heavy evening meals and alcohol at dinner time. On the other hand, a meal rich in carbohydrates with low levels of protein or fat tends to promote sleep by stimulating the production of melatonin and serotonin (beware of acidobasic imbalance). Afternoon exercise promotes sleep but should be avoided in the evening. According to a Stanford University (California) study, adults between the ages of 50 and 76 who suffer from moderate insomnia can improve their sleep quality by exercising regularly with moderate intensity. According to this study active subjects fell asleep more quickly and slept longer than sedentary subjects.

Since there are false ideas circulating on what constitutes a bad night, exaggerated fears about its impact can feed the vicious circle of insomnia. We should set realistic goals and avoid harbouring irrational beliefs (for example, believing that we need at least eight hours of sleep a night) and dramatizing the consequences of having a bad night.

Insomnia often results from bad habits. It could be that by going to bed late for some period we cause our biological clock to become desynchronized. By provoking sleep deprivation we can obtain a deeper, more regular sleep that is once more in-synch with our other biological rhythms.

These rhythms can be resynchronized by going to bed and getting up at fixed times. Sleep requirements should be adequately defined, and your bedtime should be in-synch with your waking time. It is especially the latter that regulates biological rhythm. Our bedtime should keep us somewhat sleep deprived. Let's suppose, for example, that you retire at midnight and get up at seven when you've previously determined that you need eight hours of sleep. In that case you will probably sleep deeper. If you sleep well, you should retire fifteen minutes earlier for a week, and then add fifteen minutes the next week until the required number of hours of sleep is obtained. When you feel fine in the morning it means that the number of hours allocated to sleep is sufficient. Conversely, if your quality of sleep deteriorates, you should postpone your bedtime by fifteen minutes and maintain this routine. If sleep doesn't come easily, you may getting up and find something to do.

Obviously we can also relax, belch, stretch, do breathing exercises, etc. As you know, my own sleep is disrupted, especially by digestive problems, mostly gas build-up and tension. By belching enough in the evening, I gain much in quality of sleep at night.

C – OTHER CAUSES OF ABDOMINAL PAIN

- **The genetic hypothesis** [34]

A British study reveals that patients who suffer from IBS (21% of cases) generally produce less (32 %) interleukin 10 – an anti-inflammatory substance – than the general population. In 2006, a Norwegian study conducted on twins revealed a 22% IBS concordance in the case of same-egg twins, but a mere 9% concordance when the twins were from different eggs. It is therefore possible to find a higher incidence of IBS cases in families where it is already present. Genes may than play a role, "but if IBS were purely a genetic condition, the rate of incidence among identical twins with IBS would be much higher.[35]"

- **Diet**

We know that flatulence is not only caused by air we swallow. It also results from the fermentation, in the large intestine, of foods that were undigested in the stomach and the small intestine. In fact, meal residues such as vegetable fibre require bacterial flora enzymes that produce fermentation and therefore, gas. Soluble fibres found, among other places, in apples, field berries, citrus fruits, oats, psyllium, Brussels sprouts and corn, can cause a great deal of

---

[34] Article of Mickael Bouin, gastroenterologist, « *Le syndrome de l'intestin irritable : les pistes de recherche* », *Du cœur au ventre*, AMGIF, Winter 2006, p. 3.
[35] IBS for Dummies, p. 37.

flatulence. We should also avoid eating too much insoluble fibre (such as wheat bran). These fibres can also cause dehydration of the large intestine and constipation.

In general, one should avoid gas-generating foods such as oligosaccharides or legumes (chickpeas, red kidney beans, etc.). In fact, human beings do not have the necessary enzymes to decompose the raffinose and the stachynose in beans. Moreover, some legumes are not easily digested (cabbage, broccoli, onion, turnip, radish, corn, etc.). Broccoli, Brussels sprouts, cauliflower, onions, and cabbage produce a lot odorous gas since their high sulphur content. Sodas are gaseous, although the gas they cause could be released by eructation, and into the blood stream. They apparently do not cause flatulence.

Foods that contain starch and sugar are not easily digestible and they supply the colonies of bacteria that produce gas in the large intestine. The main sugars implicated are lactose, fructose and sorbitol. Although there is little absorption through the walls of the small intestine, the bacteria moves on to the large intestine where they meet with the ones that emit CO_2, hydrogen and methane. Fructose is found in fruit juice, soda pop, apples, pears, jam and chocolate, and sorbitol in candy, plums and a number of preparations, including several medicines. A study mentioned in the book IBS for Dummies showed that one third of IBS patients were not able to digest fructose. It mentioned also that sorbitol, a sugar alcohol, acts as a fuel that bacteria use to create gas. Finally, it said that you must try to maintain your blood sugar on an even keel. Breakfast with toast, jam and a coffee saturated with sugar could increase rapidly the sugar level in your blood and so on for insulin. It could ended up, three hours later with a too low level of sugar in your blood and than making you feel dizzy and even nauseous. Concentrated fruit juices can be irritating for an IBS bowel, especially if extra sorbitol is added.

Lactose, which is found in dairy products, cannot be digested by nearly 20% of people in Western countries, because they do not possess the enzyme (lactase) that digests it. This percentage rises to 80% for African-American, Asian or Amerindian descent. Lactose malabsorption leads to diarrhoea, abdominal cramps, bloating, flatulence, etc. It can affect normal intestines or be the result of an infection, such as celiac disease. However, except for cottage cheese, most cheeses do not contain that much lactose, as in mozzarella, cheddar, brie, blue cheese, Swiss cheese, etc. When you eat dairy products, you can get lactase tablets or drops (Lactaid, for example) sold over-the-counter, or buy milk containing lower levels of lactose (Lactaid, Lacteeze, etc.).

Some people do not easily digest gluten or starch contained in flours. Gluten enteropathy occurs because the immune system attacks it using IgA and IgG antibodies. Breath tests are one of the first steps to diagnose this condition. People affected tend to have more flatulence (see chapter on celiac disease). The immune system fight means antigens and antibodies melt to neutralize antigen and to eliminate from the body by mucus from the nose, throat, urine, or stool. People[36] from Canada, Scotland and western Ireland have a higher incidence of multiple sclerosis that could be triggered by gluten intolerance. Breads, pasta and cereals should be avoided, or you can reduce this type of food in your diet, as I do. You may check whether the manufacturer has added gluten to the recipe (as in bagels) or used winter wheat, a type of wheat with higher gluten level. Rice is apparently an exception and doesn't usually cause problems.

"One study found that a group of IBS sufferers who strictly followed an elimination diet of potentially allergic foods had an 88 percent reduction in painful abdominal cramps, 90 percent elimination of diarrhoea, 65 percent less constipation, and 79 percent improvement in miscellaneous allergy symptoms. [37]"

---

[36] Ibid, p. 33.
[37] Ibid, p. 72.

Fat is known to slow down digestion and thus contribute to fermentation. It is therefore important to reduce our intake of fatty meats, sauces, cheeses with a fat content exceeding 20 %, cooked fat, fried foods, lard, pastries, etc. For example, croissants and muffins contain a substantial amount of fat, sugar and cereal. They can be especially "explosive."

Generally speaking not all of these foods cause discomfort in IBS patients. Most foods can be eaten in small amounts so that the digestive system can get used to them. However, they should not be combined with sugar, especially in the case of legumes and flour-based foods.

Your dietician can recommend a menu that will not generate gas, and your doctor can also suggest medications to relieve the pain or increase motility. Foods that generate little gas include eggs, fish, red meat, asparagus, avocado, citrus fruits, grapes, olives, tomatoes and plain yogurt. Taking walks, exercising, relaxation, strengthening your stomach muscles and drinking enough fluids will improve the circulation of gas. Finally, it is a good practice to relieve yourself when you feel the need.

If you practice gas evacuation exercises regularly, it may not be so important to radically change your dietary habits. Since it is almost impossible to stop swallowing air, evacuation exercises are a must whenever flatulence causes pain. And, as C. F. Mercier de Compiègne would say, "Get a whiff of my reasoning". My own slogan is: gas released is no longer painful!

Pharmacological treatments

Peppermint oil (Colpermin) is thought to relieve abdominal pain and bloating. It is better when the peppermint is enteric coated so that it can have an effect on the intestine. Colpermin is no longer marketed in Canada but is still available in some European countries.

Dicyclomin (Bentylol), an antispasmodic, helps relieve meteorism. It causes undesirable side-effects such as constipation, dryness of the mouth, dizziness, somnolence, visual problems and nausea.

However, it is believed to be highly effective against bloating. I turned to Dicyclomin for several years, but stopped using it as my condition improved. I would take some, for a day or two, while stress or a gastro induce stomach spasms.

You can also try α-D-galactosidase enzyme (Beano) but its effectiveness is still debated. There is also simethicone, at a maximum dosage of 540 mg per day. It seems that it reduces the pressure on the surface of gas bubbles, but it is apparently only useful when it becomes painful to pass gas. You pharmacist may recommend activated coal but its effectiveness is not proven and it can hinder drug absorption. Finally, bismuth subsalicylate (Pepto-Bismol) seems to have an effect on the sulphur-based compounds that cause the strong odour. However, medicinal interactions should limit its use.

- **Acidity**[38]

Our body naturally leans towards either acidity or alkalinity. Acidity is measured on a scale of 1 for the highest degree of acidity to 14 for the highest degree of alkalinity, 7 being the state of equilibrium. The body is equipped with a buffer system so that when it is acidified, for example, it draws alkaline minerals (calcium, magnesium, potassium and sodium) from its tissue reserves to restore balance. Eventually this may cause demineralization.

The lack of alkaline minerals or too much acidity causes the digestion of fats, sugars and proteins to be incomplete in the duodenum, which functions in an alkaline environment. Digestion must then occur deeper in the intestines, where a putrefaction process causes the smelly odour, constipation and foul-smelling stools. Conversely, too much alkalinity tends to cause bloating and often, as in my case, persistent diarrhoea.

---

[38] Hélène Baribeau, M. Sc., Dt. P., nutritionist, *Guide ressources*, November 2000, p. 24-27.

The main acidification factors are the diet, shortness of breath and a lack of physical activity. In fact, the kidneys and lungs, which are responsible for the elimination of acidity, are stimulated by deep breathing, calm and exercise. The by-products of aspirin, morphine and non-steroidal anti-inflammatory drugs (NSAID) can acidify the terrain.

Dark, coloured vegetables are alkalinizing because of their calcium, magnesium and potassium content. Non-sulphur dried fruits, avocados, potatoes, milk, corn, soy and its by-products and mild fruits (bananas, melons, pears, peaches, and apples) are also alkalinizing. Sugar, meat (proteins), some fruits (red currants, raspberries, strawberries, lemons, oranges, grapefruits, kiwis, and tomatoes), vinegar, yogurt and cheese are acid-forming.

According to nutritionist Hélène Baribeau, some plants can also help restore the balance. When the acidity is too high, the flowers of achillea, oats or camomile, raspberry's bushes leaves, alfalfa, nettle and glasswort, as well as marine algae, are often helpful. To promote the digestive process you can also try anise, dill and coriander seeds, tarragon, lemon balm, mint, oregano, thyme or rosemary, and the roots of sweet grass, angelica, chicory, ginger or rhubarb. Finally, for remineralisation you can try out oats, wheat, alfalfa, barley, nettle, parsley, dandelion, horsetail, roots of burdock, couch grass, dandelion, Jacob's-ladder, the fruits and seeds of black currants, barberry, raspberries, red currants, blackberries, blueberries; garlic cloves and marine algae.

In my point of view, the main benefit I get from these products is from the hot water I drink with them, which provides hydration and relaxes the stomach, and from the time I spend for myself as I prepare and ingest them.

To check your acidobasic equilibrium all you need to do is test the urine pH using a test-paper. It is my opinion that the companies supplying urine tests or offering food supplements to restore the acidobasic equilibrium tend to inflate the directions for use to sell more products, and post a higher price tag. The firms Kami Santé and Biosana, which sells urine tests, recommend supplements for one, and for the other, to perform the tests three times a day for three weeks. I find this is too much. My own system, for example, is alkaline and to restore its equilibrium I only need to drink one or two glasses of grapefruit juice and reduce my intake of alkaline foods, especially those that are flour based. In a single day I generally manage to restore my acidobasic equilibrium, and I can verify the results by means of the test-papers. Since in my case alkalinity causes a great deal of gas, I also have to do more evacuation exercises.

In case of an acid field, you can adjust your diet in accordance. You must then increase the intake of alkaline foods and reduce acidic foods.

I should mention that this acidobasic imbalance hypothesis and its relation to the production of gas are not acknowledged medically.

- **Food allergies** [39]

According to Dr André Caron, the incidence of true food allergies is not clear, estimates fall between 0.3 and 7.5% for children, and decrease as the child gets older.

Food pathologies can be divided into several groups. First, there are nutritional diseases related to overeating (obesity, vitamin A poisoning) or a deficiency (depression, vitamin deficiency). Then, there are undesirable food responses: poisoning (direct effect of a food, food additives or contaminants); intolerance, a reaction involving several abnormal physiological responses in predisposed individuals; food allergies or any other hypersensitivity response caused by some foods. Finally, we have the false food allergies resulting from an infection, more akin to poisoning or intolerance.

Four categories of food cause food allergies: animal, vegetable, additives and contaminants. Each can be divided into sub-groups, some of which contain several foods made up of antigenic molecules

---

[39] André Caron, M. D., *Le Clinicien*, Octobre 1995, vol. 10, n°s 10-11.

(giving rise to antigens). Some foods and pollens combine to create the same antigens, such as ragweed pollen combined with melon and banana, wormwood pollen combined with celery, birch pollen with apple, for instance.

The foods most often involved in an immediate allergic reaction are peanuts, nuts, eggs milk, soy, fish, seafood, bananas and chicken. Antigenic food molecules are generally glycoproteins that have a specific molecular weight (between 10,000 and 40,000 daltons), and are usually heat and enzyme resistant (proteolytics).

Few known foods have been studied from the point of view of their antigenic molecules. Among those most often studied are milk, eggs, peanuts and fish. Out of the 25 milk proteins, beta-lactoglobulin is the most allergenic, and its antigen is little altered by heat. Then, there is casein, which is also heat resistant, lactalbumin and bovine blood proteins that are heat sensitive (albumin and globulin). Penicillin and other substances can contaminate milk and cause reactions in some people.

Ovalbumin and ovomucoid are the main egg white antigens, and their antigenicity is not altered by cooking. Conalbumin is also antigenic. Although rare, allergies to egg proteins sometimes occur.

It seems that there are two major peanut globulins, the arachin and the conarchin, which contain several antigenic molecules; their antigenicity persists even after the peanuts are roasted.

The main allergenic component of fish is the M allergen, a parvalbumin controlling the movement of calcium in cells. Antigen II, also heat resistant, seems to be the main allergen in shrimp and shellfish.

In newborns the intestine is highly permeable to antigenic macromolecules, but this characteristic wanes rapidly after birth. Antigenic macromolecules encounter a number of defence mechanisms before reaching the digestive membrane. These molecules may then find their way into lymphoid cells or the venous blood flow and reach the liver.

People who develop an immune response to a given molecule possess the genes allowing for such a response when exposed to the antigen in question. The quantity of antigen, the exposure route, the time and length of the exposure, even the presence of an infectious disease can all affect the immune response.

It is believed that most allergic reactions to foods are related to reactions involving the immunoglobulin E (IgE). Among other things these responses cause peripheral vasodilatation, increase capillary permeability and contract the smooth muscles (especially in the bronchial tube).

True food allergies are rare. What we generally see are *food intolerances* (a term we should use instead of *allergies*) or functional digestive disorders, whose cause can often be traced to a specific food type. From there it is easy to blame a particular food or try to find a miracle diet.

- **Food intolerance** [40]

Food intolerance is an abnormal reaction to some foods (cheese, yeast extract, avocado, banana, shallot, raspberry, black currant, ginger, almonds, apricots, oranges, honey, olives, tomatoes, cashew nuts) or beverages (coffee, chocolate, tea, soda pop with caffeine, red wine). Food intolerance can also be caused by spices (curry powder, paprika, thyme, rosemary, oregano, cumin, mustard seed, anise, sage, Cayenne pepper, cinnamon, dill, allspice) or food additives (tartrazine, sodium benzoate, sulphites, monosodium glutamate, and aspartame).

The symptoms, which do not involve the immune system, usually appear several hours after eating, and their intensity is generally

---

[40] Article of Jacinthe Côté, Dietitian, « *Une allergie que l'on appelle "intolérance"* », *Le Soleil*, mars 20th 2005, p. A 13.

proportional to the concentration of the irritating agent and the quantity ingested. People who are food intolerant can often withstand some dose of the agent before the response sets in. The symptoms can appear on the skin, mouth, throat, stomach, in the digestive tract. In comparison, food allergies involve an immune response and can be triggered by the smallest amount of food. In cases of food intolerance the food to blame can often be identified by elimination. Generally, all we need to do is reduce our intake of the culprit.

• **Monosodium glutamate**

Monosodium glutamate (MSG), a natural product, is an exitotoxin that acts on the brain to make you think something tastes better. But, like aspartame, it can "overstimulate the brain causing neurons to die from exhaustion."[41] Japanese researchers have discovered a glutamate-specific receptor (or *umami*) on the tongue. Until now it was generally agreed that all the flavours came from our perception of the salty, sweet, acid or bitter. On the other hand, 15% of people cannot identify the specific taste of glutamate. An impressive quantity of foods and food additives contain MSG. Marketed under the brand name Accent, it is also a natural salt found in tomatoes, milk and mushrooms. The human body contains approximately 12 grams of it.

Although it has not been scientifically proven, glutamate can cause reactions in 1.8% of the population. Patients complain of migraine, acute arachin, burning sensations on the skin, forearms and chest combined with redness and heat in the face or nausea, a feeling of oppression, and pins and needles and dizzy spells that can occur from a few minutes to an hour following ingestion. It can also indispose asthma sufferers, cause irritability, depression, paranoia, verbal incoherence. Since MSG is largely used in prepared Chinese food these reactions are known as the "Chinese restaurant syndrome." It metabolizes very quickly in the bloodstream. Since alcohol increases

---

[41]   IBS for Dummies, p. 80.

the speed with which food is absorbed the symptoms are generally quicker and more intense with alcohol.

In 1969, Dr John W. Olney of the University of Washington reported that in some cases and at given concentrations glutamate could cause acute necrosis of the nerve cells in laboratory mice. The makers of baby foods therefore removed it from their preparations. However, in general the industry considers that at normal concentrations glutamate is harmless for adults. If there is a reaction, however, it is recommended to limit its ingestion and dilute it by drinking lots of water. If MSG is not mentioned, it can hide in the label "hydrolyzed protein." In my case, since I tend to react rather strongly to the substance, I follow these previous recommendations successfully.

• Aspartame [42]

Aspartame is produced by combining two neurotransmitters – aspartate and phenylalanine – with methanol, a wood alcohol. Methanol is freed in the small intestine where it can be transformed in formic acid and formaldehyde, which is a serious neurotoxin. Research indicates that most methanol you should consume in one day is 7.8 milligrams while one litre or pint of diet soda contains about 56 milligrams of methanol.

• Two weeks plan

The book IBS for Dummies recommends a two week plan to identify food triggers. For two weeks you must eliminate alcohol, coffee, dairy, food additives and diet products with aspartame, fried foods, fruit, corn syrup, processed foods, spicy foods, sugar and wheat of your diet. This will let time to your immune system to settled down and eliminate inflammatory and irritation responses. Fresh meats, poultry, fish, vegetables, nuts and seeds,

---

[42] Ibid, p. 317

unprocessed oils, whole grains (rice, millet, quinoa, amaranth and kasha), water, lemonade and herbal teas are allowed. Afterward you can reintroduce trigger foods one by one each day to see if your immune system reacts. If no reaction you can continue to consume that food. Gas and bloating could increase fast after an unfriendly food is ingested. If you have an allergy to a food that you've added back, you'll probably experience a rash, stuffy sinuses and/or headaches. If you have a reaction, you must wait two to three days before reintroducing another food.

- **Diverticule** [43]

Acute diverticular sigmoiditis is a rare complication occurring in people who are bearers of diverticules. Surgery and diet generally play a role in its treatment and prevention.

Diverticulosis, which means being in the presence of a diverticulum, affects approximately 5% of people who are forty years old, 30% of sixty year olds and 65% of eighty year olds. This condition consists of small hernias that develop on the walls of the colon and can become blocked or create inflammation. If a complication occurs the diverticulum can cause a haemorrhage or infection (sigmoiditis). This is the main cause of the bleeding. The bleeding generally disappears after a few days. The inflammation is often painful and accompanied by fever. If it persists it can evolve into peritonitis or perforation. Complications occur mostly with relatively young patients (under fifty).

However, diverticuli should not be mistaken for polyps, which grow inside the colon and can become cancerous. Contrary to infected diverticuli, polyps are painless. They can be diagnosed only by means of a colonoscopy.

---

[43] Renaud Leberherr, *E-santé* : http://www.e-sante.fr
Didier Loiseau, M. D., *La diverticulose*, Erda.
« *Les maladies de l'appareil digestif* », *Clinique Mayo*, Lavoie et Broquet, p. 163-171.
Article of Pierre Poitras, Gastroenterologist, *Du cœur au ventre*, AMGIF, vol. 4, n° 4, Winter 2004.

In Western societies the relative absence of fibre in the diet promotes diverticulosis. A diet low in fibre reduces the volume and hydration of stools, making their progression difficult, which destabilizes colon motility. This leads to hyperpressure zones that promote the onset of diverticuli. In the absence of inflammation, a diet with high fibre content, combined with sufficient hydration, reduces the risk of developing diverticules by lowering the internal pressure of the colon. If the diverticuli are inflamed or infected it is best to reduce the stool volume so that the colon can rest. A fibre-free diet, known as a "residue-free" diet, is then recommended. We should point out that there is no scientific basis to the fear of eating seeds, which allegedly cause inflammation by making their way into the diverticuli.

In a case of acute sigmoiditis emergency surgery is rarely contemplated. Antibiotics associated with total fast for a few days generally helps get rid of the infection. If necessary, surgery can be performed when the infection is over. In some cases antibiotics have to be prescribed for nearly a month, or intra-abdominal abscesses have to be drained under *scanner* monitoring. Some infections require emergency surgery, especially when a perforation is suspected.

The first test is an X-ray of the colon following an enema using an X-ray visible product. The other test is a colonoscopy, which helps detect other pathologies such as polyps or cancer in its early stages. In an emergency, a *scan* may be ordered to detect infectious lesions (abscesses). When there is a recurrence it is often more serious and may require emergency surgery.

• Helicobacter pylori [44]

The *Helicobacter pylori (Hp)* infection occurs when a person drinks water or eats food contaminated by human feces containing the bacteria.

It is estimated that from 50 to 80% of adults all over the world are bearers of *Hp* at the age of twenty-five, and from 60 to 70% after the age of sixty. *Hp* penetrates the gastric mucous membrane to prevent the harmful effects of stomach acid. A duodenal ulcer is present in only 15% of patients infected. Conversely, from 90 to 95% of patients who have a duodenal ulcer, and approximately 70 to 80% of patients who have a gastric ulcer are infected, the other gastric ulcers often being caused by non-steroidal anti-inflammatory drugs (NSAID). *Hp* can also cause type-B gastric lymphomas which can be treated by eliminating the bacteria. The cases of functional dyspepsia and gastroesophageal reflux do not appear to be connected with *Hp*.

The bacteria produce urease, which transforms urea into ammoniac thus raising the pH of the environment. Urease exerts a cytotoxic action liable to injure epithelial cells. It also produces CO_2 by its action on urea, a substance naturally present in the stomach. Once it has settled in, *Hp* develops proteins to mobilize and activate inflammatory cells.

Some 50% of patients suffering from peptic ulcer present epigastric burns that may last for several weeks, interrupted with periods of at least a month when the patient is symptom-free. Therefore, the

---

[44] Articles of Robert Bailey, M. D., of Naoki Chiba, M. D., of Keith G. Tolman, M. D., of Richard N. Fedorak, M. D., of Stephen Wolman, M. D., of Stepen Sontag, M. D. And of Pamela Rose, RN, B. Sc., *Le Clinicien*, STA Communications, Supplement November 1995.
Chrystian Dallaire, M. D., « *Helicobacter au pylori* », *Le Clinicien*, STA Communications, vol. 1, n° February 1996, p. 114-129.
Bernard Edmond-Jean, M. D., « *Helicobacter pylori et ulcères gastro-duodénaux* », *Le Clinicien*, STA Communications, vol. 11, n° 12, December 1996, p. 63-78.

test to detect the presence of *Hp* should take place only when the patients' symptoms are serious enough to warrant barium meal or endoscopic tests. Several tests are available to detect the bacteria: endoscopy with biopsy, serology (drop of blood), and the urea breath test, very useful in determining whether this is a recurrence (*Hp* produces urease). Endoscopy is also used to check the condition of the mucous membrane to detect lymphoma, among others. However, the urease test is faster.

In 1992, Dr Naoki Chiba indicated, in the *American Journal for Gastroenterology*, that these bacteria were eradicated by monotherapy in 18.6% of cases, by double therapy in 48.2% of cases and by triple therapy in 82% of cases. Other studies have shown that the quadruple therapy gave results approaching 95%. The treatment used to eliminate the *Hp* bacteria must generally be given to all ulcer sufferers. Here are the various proposed therapies (generally lasting seven days):

Table IV		
Treatment name	**Medication**	**Success rate**
Triple therapy with proton pump inhibitor (European approach)	Omeprazole with clarithromycine and metronidazole or amoxicilline	85 à 95%
Bismuth triple therapy (American approach)	Bismuth with tetracycline or amoxicilline and metronidazole	85 à 90%
Quadruple therapy	Omeprazole with bismuth tetracycline and metronidazole	95%

Surgery is not a frequent option in a case of uncomplicated duodenal ulcers. However, it is advisable in cases of heavy haemorrhaging or perforation. As there is a real possibility that a vaccine will eventually be developed, this disease could become rare in the Western world.

• Inflammatory diseases

Before talking about inflammatory diseases we should mention a study by Dr O'Sullivan[45] showing that tissue mass cells, which are inflammatory cells, were found more often in the colon of patients suffering from IBS than in others. In 2000, Dr Salvik from New Zealand confirmed these results in his survey of 77 patients with IBS, in addition to finding other inflammatory cells in half of them (lymphocydes in the mucus membrane) and neutrophiles (40% of cases). According to the 1998 Bearcroft study, there is a higher serotonin secretion in patients suffering from IBS with diarrhœa, especially after meals. Serotonin has a strong influence on secretion, motility and digestive sensitivity. Moreover, a British study has shown that patients suffering from IBS generally produce less Interleukin 10, an anti-inflammatory substance, than the general population.

Ulcers and anxiety [46]

Formerly, gastrointestinal ulcers were treated by focusing especially on the *helicobacter pylori* bacteria. Today, the cause of this ailment is also investigated from a psychological standpoint. Anxiety disorders and ulcers do seem to be connected.

This relationship was found to exist in people between the ages of 15 to 54. The authors of a research found that there was a connection between response and level. The mechanism has not yet been identified, but a number of hypotheses were considered: the influence of anxiety on ulcer development, or vice-versa, the possibility that ulcers could generate an anxiety disorder; an environmental or genetic factor governing the two diseases.

---

[45] Mickael Bouin, Gastroenterologist, « *Le syndrome de l'intestin irritable : les pistes de recherche* », *Du cœur au ventre*, AMGIF, Winter 2006, p. 2-3.

[46] Isabelle Eustache, M. D., *E-santé*, from an article of Renée D. Goodwin, Psychosomatic Medicine, November-December 2002.

However, researchers generally consider that people who suffer from anxiety tend to evoke symptoms associated with gastroduodenal ulcers. General anxiety apparently affects the body's immune response to bacterial infection, including *Hp* infections. Even though this study has its limits, it suggests that the patients' care should be twofold and combine anti-infectious treatments and tranquillizers.

Researchers know that twice as much IBS patients have symptoms of anxiety, panic attacks and depression[47]. Sometimes doctors will prescribe antidepressants to block the perception of pain. Tofranil will cause constipation and the serotonin reactive uptake inhibitors such as Prozac appear to cause more diarrhoea. In 2002, a group of ten U.S. gastroenterologist from the American College of Gastroenterology (the ACG group) were given the task of reviewing the current status of effective treatments for IBS. The group found that the tricyclic antidepressants, like Tofranil, were no more effective than a placebo for relieving all IBS symptoms. But the drugs did relieve IBS abdominal pain.

Celiac disease [48]

Dr Sanders and his colleagues conducted a survey with 300 patients suffering from IBS. They systematically applied to them a diagnostic procedure designed for celiac disease (gliadine IgG and IgA antibodies, anti-endomysial antibodies). The results were compared with those obtained with 300 healthy subjects. The team also performed biopsies among the patients who revealed the presence of antibodies. In all, 66 patients had positive antibodies and 14 patients, or 4.7%, had celiac disease. Among the other 52

---

[47] Ibid. pp. 148 and 158-159.
[48] *Science*, 297 : 2275-9, 2002 : http://www.sciencemag.org/
E-santé : http://www.e-sante.fr
Wahnschaffe Gastroenterology 2001;121:1329-1338 and Sanders DS and coll. *Lancet* 2001; 358 : 1504-8, medical review online *Agora* : http://www.agora.fr
« *Les maladies de l'appareil digestif* », *Clinique Mayo*, Lavoie and Broquet, chap. IX, p. 149-161 : www.broquet.qc.ca

patients, 9 were no longer heard of or refused the biopsy and the remaining 43 had a normal duodenal mucous membrane. Only 2 out of the 66 who had antibodies were found to have the disease. The authors conclude that IBS is linked significantly to celiac disease. Under these circumstances doctors may recommend that people who suffer from IBS be tested for celiac disease. Moreover, considering the large number of people having specific gluten-related antibodies, it would be to their advantage to try a gluten free diet, or at least reduce their gluten intake substantially, which is what I do.

Celiac disease causes malabsorption of foods resulting from an inflammation, and even the disappearance of villi in the small intestine's mucous membrane. Without these the body cannot absorb several essential nutriments. The patients have symptoms of diarrhoea, abdominal gas and bloating, frequent fatigue, weight loss, stunted growth in children, and premature osteoporosis. Celiac disease can be accompanied by mood swings, joint pain, muscle cramps, skin rashes, oral abscesses, tingling sensations in the legs, and numbness.

The disease is caused by the toxicity of the gluten, particularly one of its peptides, the alpha-gliadine. This discovery was made by scientists from the Stanford and Oslo universities who isolated this peptide, whose specific immune response-triggering action was demonstrated in patients with celiac disease. They also discovered that peptidase, an enzyme that digests some proteins, could help treat celiac disease caused by gliadine, which is a part of the gluten. Dr Khosla and his colleagues exposed the gliadine to various enzymes *in vitro* on rat and human tissues. However, it will be several more years before peptidase supplements are available to treat patients with celiac disease, even if these experiments are conclusive on humans.

In general the diagnosis is confirmed by a blood test called "antitransglutaminase antibody." At this time, the only effective treatment for the disease is a gluten free diet. A complete cure generally requires several months, even two to three years. A French study has shown that on average, only 10% of the foods found in grocery stores are gluten-free. According to the *Mayo Clinic* the following foods do not contain any gluten: innards, butter, margarine, vegetable oil, coffee, spices, herbs, cheese, fruits, milk, vegetables, legumes, corn, eggs, pepper, potatoes, rice, salt, soy, sugar, tea and herbal tea, tofu, meat, poultry, fish, shellfish, wine, port, cider, sake, yogurt (except yogurt containing starch). The authors of IBS for Dummies suggest using Stonyfield Farms products for the right kind of yogurt.

According to a study published in the *Wahnschaffe Gastroenterology* journal (2001; 121 : 1329-1338), nearly a third of all patients suffering from IBS along with diarrhoea are gluten intolerant, as are those suffering from celiac disease. However, even with the help of a gluten-free diet the diarrhoea and biological symptoms were not alleviated so much in patients with irritable bowels but no biological signs of celiac disease.

We can therefore conclude that some patients with IBS should contemplate, or at least try out, a diet low in gluten. Cereals with little gluten are millet, quinoa, buckwheat and amaranth. A low gluten diet is very different from the Canadian and American diets. In the near future we may see bread made from wheat, rye, kamut or spelt wheat that would be well tolerated. The gluten in these breads would be pre-digested by specific lactobacillus bacteria. As patients with IBS wait for peptidase tablets to be available, a diagnostic test could help rule out celiac disease and determine whether a gluten-free diet would be suitable in their case.

Crohn's disease [49]

Every year, two new cases of Crohn's disease add to the twenty to forty people suffering from the disease, in a population of one hundred thousand. Crohn's disease occurs most frequently in Caucasians who are natives of Europe or North America. It generally affects men and women between the ages of 15 and 35. Although not associated with IBS, Crohn's disease can however occur at the same time.

Crohn's disease is characterized by a chronic inflammation of the digestive system. The cases can be roughly divided into three thirds: a third involves only the large intestine, another third, the small intestine and the last one, the intestines as a whole. However, the disease can also affect the upper digestive system causing nausea, vomiting and pain in the pit of the stomach (epigastralgia). The symptoms of this auto-immune inflammation are diarrhoea and abdominal pain, often accompanied by weight loss, fatigue, fever and rectal discomfort. The disease evolves by bouts and can lead to ulcers.

In 2004, a study showed that a microbacterium (*mycobacterium avium subspecies paratuberculosis*) is linked to the disease. The authors found that this bacterium is present in half of the patients suffering from Crohn's disease, and in 20% of the subjects with haemorrhagic colitis, whereas it is missing in the control subjects. These results, although preliminary, suggest that some may be treatable with antibiotics.

---

[49] Article *L'origine bactérienne se confirme, E-santé*, by Dr Philippe Presles, Octobre 6th 2004, from an article of Naser S. A. et coll., *The Lancet*, 2004, 364 : 1039-1044.
S. B. Hanauer, *Maladies inflammatoires de l'intestin*, In Nennett J.-C. et coll. « *Cecil – Traité de médecine interne* » – 1st French edition, Flammarion, *Médecine-Sciences*, Paris, 1997 : 707-715.
Traitement des maladies inflammatoires de l'intestin, GNP – Encyclopédie pratique du médicament 2000, Éditions du Vidal, Paris, 1999, p. 616-620.
Les maladies de l'appareil digestif, Clinique Mayo, Lavoie et Broquet, p. 129-148.

The walls of the intestines can be affected in different areas: if the whole depth of the wall is affected it will crack and become ulcerous causing it to bleed. The affected areas will then scar and become fibrous, thereby reducing the intestine's ability to absorb foods and causing it to narrow.

It is crucial to maintain a proper diet with low fibre content (no fibrous fruits and vegetables) especially where diarrhoea is present, and low fat content. The vitamin intake should be closely watched.

Over the years many complications could surface. The most common is bowel obstruction (caused by stricture) and cancer of the digestive tract (including the colon), justifying the rather frequent use of colonoscopy. A blood test and an X-ray of the small intestine and of the colon can also help make a diagnosis.

The treatments relieve the symptoms but they do not bring about a cure. They consist mainly in mesalazine suppositories or enemas (Pentasa, Rowasa), and cortisone derivatives administered by enema (Betnesol, Rectovalone), rectal foam (Colofoam, Proctocort), or systemically (by mouth or injection). In some cases the cortisone treatment must be permanent. Immunosuppressants are also useful in some cases. Anti-diarrheics, laxatives, analgesics and iron or vitamin supplements are also largely used.

One out of two patients is operated on to remove a portion of the intestine of varying size when there are very frequent attacks – poorly controlled by medication – of heavy bleeding, intestinal blockage or threat of blockage, suspicion of cancer, etc. It is estimated that 50 % of patients who had surgery will need another surgery, and so on.

However, at the end of the day it appears that the effectiveness of local treatments (mesalazine and cortisone), and the advances in the field of surgery have helped extend the life of patients suffering from Crohn's disease. Finally, if the hypothesis of a bacterial infection is confirmed, an antibiotic treatment can be a promising avenue.

- **Stomach cancer** [50]

Stomach cancer is rare and its incidence is not IBS related. It can be treated while the tumour is still superficial. Surgery remains the most appropriate treatment. Risk factors include salt and nitrites. Some cancers appear to result from an infection caused by *helicobacter pylori*.

Only surgery to remove a large part of the stomach can bring about a cure. Chemotherapy can be used as a palliative treatment, or to help reduce the size of the tumour to allow surgery to be performed.

As opposed to cancer of the oesophagus, stomach cancer in its early stages does not hinder the ingestion of foods. Its first signs are an ulcer, which can be painful or bleed, and weight loss. To examine the stomach, the gastroenterologist will use oesogastric fibroscopy. A sample is removed to detect the presence of cancerous tissue. A scan of the abdomen will determine if the cancer has spread to the lymph nodes and neighbouring organs, and if metastases are present in the liver.

- **Benign and malignant tumours of the colon** [51]

Benign tumours of the colon mainly consist of polyps or protrusions ranging in sizes from 2mm to several centimetres. There are two types of benign colon tumours: hyperplastic polyps, which can never develop into cancer, and adenomatous polyps which can. In France, 5 to 10% of people over the age of 45 present adenomatous polyps, and of these, 5 to 10% will develop cancer. These adenomatous polyps cause 75% of all colon cancers. It takes an average of five to ten years for an adenoma to turn malignant. Colon cancer affects approximately 5% of the population.

---

[50] Renaud Guichard, M. D., *E-santé* : http://www.e-sante.fr_
[51] From an article in Web magazine *Médisite* : http://www.medisite.fr/
    Philippe Presles, M. D., *E-santé*, from an article « Cancer Epidemiology,
    Biomarkers & Prevention », 13 : 1253-1256, 2004; *Journal of the National
    Cancer Institut*, 2004, 96 : 1015-1022.
    Article of Pierre Poitras, Gastroenterologist, *Du cœur au ventre*, AMGIF,
    vol. 4, n° 4, Winter 2004.

There is no link between IBS and colon cancer. Upon examination some signs can point to this type of cancer: recent pain, changes in stool patterns especially after fifty years old, blood in the stools. Like all cancers it can be divided into four stages. In the first stage it is small and limited to the intestine with no lymph nodes or metastases. It is 100% curable by surgery. The last stage involves damage to organs located in other parts of the body, such as the liver. At that stage only 5 to 15% of patients are likely to survive after five years, hence the importance of an early diagnosis.

The role of heredity in some forms of colorectal cancer has been suspected for quite a while. A Swedish survey conducted with over ten million people confirmed that the brothers and sisters of people with this type of cancer are up to seven times more likely to develop it. We should keep in mind that environmental factors are important. For example, an international study showed that the consumption of milk products reduces the risk of suffering from this type of cancer. The cells lining the walls of the digestive tract are the first to be in contact with the food we eat, and they are known to renew themselves rapidly, which explains the risk of polyps that can sometimes turn into malignant tumours. According to a team of British researchers, 80% of cancers of the digestive tract can be traced to a poor diet. The existence of an inflammatory intestinal disease, as well as dietary habits, apparently increases its occurrence.

Polyps are rarely symptomatic, except when they are large. Bleeding through the lower part of the body (rectorrhagia) or abdominal pain can then occur. During a clinical examination the doctor palpates the lymph node areas and makes a rectal examination, which can reveal a polyp, or rectal haemorrhoids. A stool sample analysis may show traces of blood. The doctor will then turn to colonoscopy to have a look at the tumour and perform a biopsy. Most of the time polyps can be removed by colonoscopy. Older people should see their doctor when rectorrhagia is present, and not be content with a hemorrhoid diagnosis.

The cancer prognosis depends on the stage of discovery of the disease. When a polyp is removed by endoscopy it is considered a cure. A cancer discovered in a locally limited area is easier to treat. Polyp and cancer cases require the regular monitoring of the colon.

Cancers of the digestive tract are also easy to prevent by adopting a diet with a high fruit and vegetable content, rich in folate (folic acid or vitamin B$_9$), polyunsaturated fat and flavonoids (antioxidants). On the other hand, a recent review of the literature contradicts the assumption that food fibre helps prevent these cancers.

Colonoscopy is the most accurate test. It generally allows for an immediate treatment and it is good for approximately ten years. It is a relatively expensive test and there are long waiting lists, at least in Canada. However, it should be considered when blood is found in the stools, when there is an incriminating family history, or a doubt persists and the patient is over fifty. A barium enema or a sigmoidoscopy – a procedure not as expensive but less accurate – can be performed. In any case, if doctor's doubt persists colonoscopy is a must.

• **Physiological particularities**

Dr Mickael Bouin, gastroenterologist, presented results of a study showing that the majority of people with IBS have their diaphragm 1cm (half an inch) lower than those without IBS. This could pressure the upper part of the large intestine making gas passage more difficult. I try to correct this by deep breathing with an upward move of my ribs. I also posture my ribs higher when in my bed so that less pressure is made on the upper part of my large intestine. This favours gas passage in the large intestine. If, like me, you work seated all day, you're also at risk of blocking bloat passage. In my case, I'm always bloated after work.

Some people are also short-waisted.[52] If you have less than 5 inches between your last rib and your hipbone, you are short-waisted and

---

[52] IBS for Dummies, p. 27.

there is less room for your 20 feet of intestine to accommodate gas passage.

D) – RECENT HYPOTHESES

• The other brain

The central nervous system [53]
The central nervous system (CNS) plays a major role in the digestive system's equilibrium. It can tell us that we urgently need to go, but also help us hold it in, so that we can relieve ourselves in the proper place. During stressful periods it has an impact on the digestive system by its action on hormones and neurotransmitters. For some it has an effect on the stomach, in others it accelerates (diarrhoea) or slackens (constipation) intestinal motility. People who suffer from IBS react to stress faster and with more intensity. When pain is associated with these symptoms we refer to hypersensitivity. Normally, it is the autonomous nervous system which controls the internal organs. In fact, one of its parts, the enteric nervous system, hugs the tissues of the digestive organs.

More and more scientists find that chronic disorders of the digestive system result from a complex interaction between sensitivity, the autonomous nervous system, intestinal motility and the CNS. In nearly thirty years of practice Pallardy has developed and tested on himself and on his patients a number of techniques (see the chapter on Pierre Pallardy's approach) in order to restore smooth communication between the two brains, that of the abdomen, and of the cerebral cortex.

In fact, researches tend to show that the digestive system can increasingly be compared, on the structural and neurochemical levels,

---

[53] *Participate,* International Foundation for Functional Gastrointestinal Disorders (IFFGD), vol. 7, n° 2, Summer 1998, p. 1-5, vol. 9, n° 4, Winter 2000, et vol. 11, n° 1, Spring 2002.
Pierre Pallardy, *Et si ça venait du ventre?* Robert Laffont, S. A., Paris, 2002, 257 p.

to a second brain. It produces 70 to 85% of the body's immune cells, the so-called "interstitial" cells that play a role in muscle functioning. It houses a complex network of neurotransmitters, neuromodulators and molecules that are identical to brain molecules (serotonin, melatonine, acetylcholine, epinephrine, netrin, etc.). According to Dr Michael D. Gershon of Columbia University, author of the book *The Second Brain*, our two brains, in our head and in our abdomen, must co-operate, otherwise it leads to chaos for our abdomen and misery for our head. They discovered, among other things, that some elements involved in Alzheimer's disease and Parkinson's are also found in the digestive system.

Occasionally, a psychological problem such as a trauma, a depression, a panic disorder or a food disorder, may cause problems similar to those resulting from IBS. For a long time researchers have noted that some antidepressants reduced the digestive tract's sensitivity. At low doses they are now prescribed for many patients with IBS. In the United States antidepressants have been used to treat IBS for almost forty years. It is believed that in some people nervous cells are more or less resistant to norepinephrin and serotonin. Over the years there are less of these substances in the cells, which can lead to depression and greater sensitivity to pain. Although several types of antidepressants have been used to treat IBS, the ones prescribed most often are medicines that act on serotonin inhibitors such as Prozac, Luvoz or Paxil. This type of antidepressants is also used in the treatment of anxiety disorders, obsessive-compulsive disorders and post-traumatic shocks.

In 1987, Dr Greenbaum and colleagues showed that antidepressants are helpful in IBS cases, even when psychic disorders are not involved. Dr Richard O. Cannon had discovered that another type of antidepressant, imipramme, relieved symptoms of oesophageal dismotility (chest pains not resulting from cardiac disorders). Dr M. Handa and colleagues discovered that Paxil also provided relief in these cases. Today, Quebec and France are the places where the highest number of antidepressants is prescribed throughout the Western world.

There are several types of serotonin: 5-HT1 and 5-HT2, with concentration in the brain, and 5-HT3 and 5HT4, mostly found in the intestines. Nowadays researches involve medicines that have an impact on these types of serotonin, and on IBS treatment, without falling into the antidepressant category. This is the case with Zelnorm, a medication mostly prescribed to women, which acts on a specific type of serotonin receptor (type 4). It is also prescribed to men suffering from chronic constipation and for people suffering from IBS and constipation. Due to complications for few patients, Zelnorm have been withdrawn.

In general, patients are prescribed antidepressants to relieve the symptoms of IBS. The depression-causing aspect of IBS is a difficult problem and there is a risk of addiction that must be closely managed. Antidepressants must be part of a detailed approach to the IBS treatment, in collaboration with a health care professional.

When other approaches have failed, psychotherapy, whether or not it is associated with a medication, can reduce IBS symptoms. The most commonly used therapies are those of the cognitive type, these deal with upsetting external events, help improve living conditions or manage the major symptoms. Techniques used to manage stress, relaxation and hypnosis, are also known for their ability to reduce the intensity and occurrence of digestive disorders. Another interesting and low-cost avenue may be abdominal breathing, which solicits both the brain (will) and relaxation of the abdomen (the other brain) in an effort to harmonize the two brains.

Chronic pain

Even when chronic pain is not an element of the IBS diagnosis, most surveys show that some 60% of patients indicate that it is among their symptoms. Most of these patients have a high degree of visceral sensitivity. Yet the pain associated with FDDs are usually more diffuse than muscle pain or superficial wounds, for instance. Researchers conducted on chronic pain tend to indicate that it is a pathology of the nervous system and an inadequate response of the brain and spinal cord.

Pain is an element of survival. It warns us that we have been injured, it allows us to move away from danger (withdrawal reflex), forces us to take a rest (to look after ourselves or allow the pain to subside), protect ourselves (so as not to make the pain worse); move away, even warns others of the danger (cry). The underlying physiological basis of normal pain appears to be the same as for chronic pain. A person who suffers from chronic pain has the impression that the hurt is constant.

According to Dr Bruce D. Naliboff, from 30 to 40 million Americans experience chronic pain for more than six months. Chronic pain is the main reason why people consult their doctors. Dr John Liebeskind of the University of California at Los Angeles (UCLA) is one of the first scientists who showed that persistent pain is detrimental to the immune system. Animals that were inoculated with a cancer lived longer if they were given morphine to alleviate the pain.

The pain associated with FDDs covers two major avenues: a cellular alteration of the gastric and intestinal wall and a problem in the modulation of exchanges of the nervous system in communicating the pain. These are the same avenues involved in chronic pain researches.

Medication used to relieve chronic pain gives good results in some fields such as the cases of pain associated with inflammation. Several pain relieving medicines are derivatives of antidepressants or anticonvulsants. However, chronic pain often has to be treated with narcotics or opiates, which can lead to tolerance and create addiction. These medications must be well managed to avoid the continuous increase in dosage and ensure that the patient remains functional.

According to Dr Naliboff an active approach (exercise, information taking, and preventing potential deterioration) generally appears to produce better results than a passive or dependent approach in the patient to doctor relationship. The patient must pay special attention to sources of stress (fatigue, irritability, insomnia, loss of concentration and interest). He or she should also undertake relaxation techniques, exercise regularly and develop a positive yet realistic attitude. For example, patients should avoid thinking about catastrophic scenarios. During difficult periods they should recall that they've lived through such periods before, or try to find new treatment options. The efforts should be centered on what can be changed or influenced. In this connection, making sure that sleeping conditions are optimal can be a solution. To avoid a tendency towards isolation, patients should try to join in social activities even though they may not feel like it. These activities can provide support or unsuspected referrals. Alternative medicines are also an option. However, few scientific studies have proved their effectiveness. A consultation in a specialized chronic pain management clinic can be a good investment in cases of chronic pain.

The signs of trauma [54]

Some studies link IBS with work, money, couple, shelter, social relations problems. Dr Ghislain Devroede, a colorectal surgeon and a professor at Sherbrooke University, was one of the first to establish a connection between FDDs and sexual abuse, especially in early childhood. He considers himself to be an expert of the "fondement" (posterior), a term derived from old French and designating the perineum. According to Dr Devroede, the interactions between the urinary, sexual, reproductive and digestive functions are countless, and their complexity is underestimated because the scientific approach underlying the concept of "fondement" is piecemeal. It is also to Dr Devroede's credit that he developed an "integrated vision of the abdomen, of the "fondement" and of their interactions with the mind and the past" (p. 13). According to him, the medical and

---

[54] Ghislain Devroede, *Ce que les maux de ventre disent de notre passé*, Paris, Payot, February 2003, 311 p.
David Servan-Schreiber, M. D. et psychiatre, *Guérir le stress, l'anxiété et la dépression sans médicaments ni psychanalyse*, Robert Laffont, Paris, 2003, 302 p.

surgical approaches are not effective in treating FDDs. He notes that, "psychotherapy is the only way to reduce the pain, abdominal bloating and diarrhoea" (p. 20). His argumentation regarding the unfortunate contradiction between the psychological, physiological and scientific approaches is highly rewarding.

Almost 15 % of IBS patients treated by gastroenterologists suffer from deep depression. Sometimes treating depression is enough to alleviate IBS related complains. Depression is known to slow intestinal transit while anxiety speeds it. For example, hyperventilation while patient suffers anxiety tends to make him or her more sensitive to abdominal pain. In his book entitled "Guérir le stress, l'anxiété et la dépression sans médicaments ni psychanalyse" ("Curing stress, anxiety and depression without medication or psychoanalysis"), Dr David Servan-Schreiber, psychiatrist, develops the in-depth notion of an emotional brain. The architecture, cellular make-up and biochemical properties of this brain are not the same as the neocortex's, a part of the brain particularly developed in humans. The emotional brain controls a person's psychological well-being, as well as a great deal of the body's physiology. Emotional disorders are the result of a dysfunction of the emotional brain, itself the result of past painful experiences. These experiences continue to control the way we feel things and our behaviour. The psychotherapist's task is to reprogram the brain so that it can adjust to the present instead of repeating the adjustments of the past. Methods that involve the body directly have an impact on the emotional brain, not language or reason, which are unable to penetrate the emotional brain. The author adds that this brain is equipped with natural self-healing mechanisms. The following section, entitled "Other exercises", describes techniques that can be used to bring together and harmonize the emotional brain and the neocortex.

When he sees a FDDs patient Dr Devroede carefully notes the words, gestures, eyes and emotions he or she expresses. He will note, for instance, the patient's tone of voice, whether there is logorrhoea (excessive talkativeness), silent constipation, stuttering, etc. He notes inappropriate behaviours that often indicate a hidden agenda or silent suffering. He also asks patients about possible phobias. Constipated phobic patients, for example, often present a high level of hysteria. He gets physically close to the patients, sometimes to the point of touching them. Hysterical personalities do not easily accept proximity or touching.

Dr Devroede suspects that several FDDs sufferers "somatise" their emotions, especially anger, rather than "mentalizing" them, which express personality dissociation. To explain why patients appear to play down the importance of unpleasant events, he suggests that instead of getting angry and dealing with the consequences of a given event they contract their colon. Such an "expression" has the advantage of being reversible. He explains that we have four ways of expressing ourselves when we are intensely affected by something. Ideally we do it through speech, emotion and tears. If speech fails us, the body takes over and speaks in a dissociative manner. When this occurs, however, one does not constructively assume the triggering events or his or her emotions. He or she may feel like a victim, therefore passive, with regard to this body that expresses itself in his or her place and gives so much trouble. The patient may then become addicted to medications or doctors.

When they see a patient, doctors closely watch for transfer situations they have learned to guard against by remaining cold or distant. Dr Devroede, for his part, tends to help patients realize to what extent their FDDs symptoms may be related to a personality disorder. He shows himself to be receptive to the anger of patients without getting involved in their emotions, a very difficult thing to do for a caregiver. In this connection, a verbal expression of anger can be a sign of progress. However, this approach is not an easy one in today's world: "Doctors who treat the body no longer seem to deal with the psyche [...] secularization has made us tip over, from a culture of transgression in which people became sick because they had sinned against God, to another culture as filled with projections as the other, the culture of prejudice in which, if the person being treated is not doing well it is the caregiver's fault. As for psychiatrists, they increasingly turn to chemical poultices to close the gaps through which suffering could emerge, aiming at the functional rather than the existential, at the short-term rather than at the long-term recovery process" (free translation p. 272-273).

While I was undergoing analysis I found that anger is often a jumble, an attempt to express difficult emotions that I would rather ignore. If anger is a bad counsellor, analysing the causes of this emotion can be particularly revealing, especially while I let myself feel the hidden emotions behind.

According to Dr Devroede, people who suffer from anism present a typical case of dissociation. The constipation related to anism is caused by bearing down to defecate and, at the same time, contracting the perineum to prevent it. "It is the body's functional signature of a dissociative process" (free translation p. 33).

The same can be said of breathing. According to Dr Devroede, subjects who have been abused are unable to breathe deeply (thoracic breathing). Others tend to hyperventilate during an endoscopic exam. He may suggest that a patient look him in the eye without interruption and follow his own rhythm of breathing: he then slows down the rhythm as much as possible while increasing its scope and depth, the same as in my own breathing technique. When he feels intuitively that a patient is ready to express a hidden emotion, Dr Devroede tells them to increase their respiratory rhythm to a maximum, as in the primal scream therapy, or holotropic breathing. This can prevent convulsions and blackouts (vagal shock), and rather than experience an anxiety attack and hyperventilation the patient often lets go and can feel deep emotional relief.

Dr Devroede's book deals at length with various types of "karma." He refers to a number of books, studies and well documented cases. There are examples of colopaths or patients who regularly experience traumas or undergo a surgical procedure. It can be an operation, but also an attack that they suffer on their birthday, when they are at the age when one of their parents became sick or suffered a trauma, or when their child is at the age when they themselves or their parents fell ill or were traumatized, etc. Sometimes a parent (up to 60% of new fathers) may become sick after the birth of a first child. This attests to the fact that psychological, social and family aspects can have an impact and, by extension, lead a surgeon who is not attuned to the patient's problems to perform avoidable surgery.

For example, he refers to a study by Dr Joséphine Hilgard, a medical doctor and psychologist, who demonstrates that there is a statistically significant link in many women, between the onsets of mental illness, the age of their oldest child and their age at the death of their mother. He points to an increasing number of published studies showing that approximately 50% of cases of women who consult a doctor for functional colopathy were the victims of sexual abuse before the age of fourteen (two thirds of the cases) and, in 90% of the cases, that the treating physician ignored it. "The abuser and the abused form an accursed alliance, and this also happen with boys" (p. 88). According to Pr Jacques Rogé, FDDs victims are often subjected to unjustified surgery. In France, 35% of patients who see their doctor for colitis had unwarranted surgery to remove their appendix. In the United States it is estimated that nearly a third of women who have had their ovaries removed were suffering from FDDs instead. In a study over 90,000 patients' records, "researchers showed that patients with IBS had three times the normal rate of gall bladder surgery and twice the rate of appendectomy and hysterectomy. IBS patients also had a 50 percent higher rate of back surgery.[55]" Another study showed that, of women consulting a gynecology clinic complaining pelvic pain, only 8 percent of women with IBS also had a true gynecological problem[56]. You must remind that if you go to a nutritionist first, you have less chance to have a surgery than if you go to a surgeon first.

Based on a personality test given to approximately one hundred colopathic patients, Dr Devroede found that these patients, more often than the control subjects, suffered from sleeping disorders, had

---

[55] IBS for Dummies, p. 97.
[56] Ibidem.

more frequent dreams and more psychopathology symptoms. Some FDDs can be better managed through a bodily approach. In cases of anism, for example, biofeedback therapy can cure on average a third of the children, improve the condition of another third without however relieving the constipation, and the last third remains dysfunctional and constipated. Biofeedback therapy seems to give better results based on the number of sessions, which suggests that there is a learning process at work here. Dr Devroede also talks about meditation as a healing tool, without however developing the topic. Of course, my exercises are not mentioned in his book.

Dr Devroede writes at length and with refinement about the therapeutic touch, noting that this type of examination stimulates the body and awakens the mind. He refers to the works of Chantal Rossignol, for whom patients "talk about their body when we would like them instead to express their emotions, but they tell their life story and release their emotions when we work on their body" (p. 245). Studies have shown that the therapeutic touch, in a lab, slows down cardiac rhythm. According to Dr Devroede, the examination must be an integral part of the therapeutic process aimed at restoring a balanced health in anyone who suffers (p. 198). Sick people who were never treated tenderly in their lives come to consider this lack as normal. During consultations, the therapeutic touch is usually limited to mechanical palpation, invasive needles or tubes inserted in their orifices. Yet, therapeutic touch is also a part of our humanity (p. 203).

Dr Devroede's book is undoubtedly one of the most interesting works on FDDs, among the most stimulating I have read on this subject to date.

Psychosomatics [57]

I believe that the symbolic interpretation of symptoms, treated extensively in literature, has more to do with an act of faith that

---

[57] Henry G. Tietze, *Votre corps vous parle, écoutez-le*, Le Jour, 1989, 211 p. (Free translation of extracts from the French version).

with sound scientific results. Since it concerns symbolism, i.e., phenomena that are at once cultural and non-measurable, there is a strong temptation to generalize. The credibility of this approach rests largely on the credibility of the authors and on the therapeutic experiments they perform. This being said, I would like to refer to a few extracts (free translation) from a text by psychotherapist Henry G. Tietze, to emphasize the importance of introspection as an activity that can contribute to self-healing. However, I recommend the greatest caution when making a connection between a symptom and its "interpretation."

Arthur Janov writes about the consequences of suppressing feelings during childhood: "This primal suffering is most often integrated into our personality so that we no longer feel it and it remains unrecognized most of the time. The system that causes us to be ill expresses this primal suffering automatically because it needs to free itself in one way or another, consciously or not. This freeing movement can occur through a smile that seems to say: "Be nice with me!" through disease meaning: "Take care of me!" or through behaviour meaning: "Look at me, dad."

What's new in this holistic approach to health is that it calls upon the notion of responsibility. According to the author life is a continuous learning process, illnesses and crises prompt us to discover what connects some disorders and behaviours and our view of things. When illness is present it is not enough to eliminate the physical symptoms, it is especially important to discover the cause of this imbalance and to find out how we can reinforce our immune system and our self-healing powers. The illness, pain and suffering incite us, through a painful release process, to break free from the goals, ideals and habits that are now obsolete, transform ourselves radically and give new meaning to our lives.

Dr Franz Alexander notes that the chronic suppression of aggressiveness, the repression and lack of expression of hostile impulses tense up the body and are related to the onset of migraines, high blood pressure, hyperthyroidism, arthritis and diabetes. The chronic inhibition of the act of asking for help (the impossibility of satisfying our desire for safety and protection) is linked to colic, exhaustion, asthma, stomach ulcer and constipation.

Diarrhoea can symbolize the desire to free ourselves from psychological pressures. In the case of constipation it could be the pressing desire not to give up in the face of an apparently insoluble problem. We may say to ourselves, "I can hold on!" In this type of situation, "you clench your teeth and your buttocks", and "plug all the openings." With muscles contracted we refuse to give in, on the sentimental as well as on the digestive level we become impenetrable and withdraw into ourselves.

Self-observation: the first step towards healing

Anyone who is tense or sick should observe, for a few weeks (I would suggest a few years), the psychosomatic connections that appear during their daily activities and write those down. It is only necessary to devote fifteen minutes a day to this exercise, note events, conversations, fights, feelings of discomfort, or the inconvenience experienced on that day. Staying tuned in allows us to bring out of its shell, "the beast" that lies dormant inside us before it is unleashed.

Tietze mentions that one of his friends was in terrible pain from nocturnal flatulence. This friend felt that he was filled with a ceaseless rage. Tietze advised him to try introspection, analyse his situation and write down his thoughts. One day the friend mentioned that he had stopped trying to fight his feelings of discomfort after realizing that his symptoms were symptoms of an anger that had been raging inside him since the beginning. This self-examination revealed that his rage was sometimes accompanied by sadness. One day he realized that ever since the birth of his son he had been experiencing an inner conflict, that although he loved him dearly he rejected him because he envied him. His infantile desire was to go back into his mother's womb.

A desire such as this may seem ridiculous in an adult, but the actual cause was of course deeply hidden in his subconscious. When he was four and his mother was pregnant with his sister he had experienced for the first time a feeling of jealousy. He felt rejected by his mother and would have liked to be back inside her womb. As this was impossible he turned his back on this desire and suppressed it. Ever since that time he had been hiding this rage in his abdomen without ever expressing it. The arousal of this desire had turned into stomach pain.

As soon as we feel symptoms we should ask ourselves: "What did I experience, think about or do today?" Answering this question in our diary can clarify the causes of our discomfort and what to do to relieve it. It also allows us to consider new avenues to help reduce and even eliminate the symptoms as well as the pain.

People who are sick generally repress all the negative emotions such as sadness, pain, fear and anger, which they often consider as weaknesses. This repression is an obstacle to their recovery, and the resulting symptoms spoil their quality of life. They are afraid they may lose all control of themselves and their environment. They perceive their body as an enemy that will not submit and agree to function properly. They appear to be unaware of parts of their experiences and realities, are unable to find their meaning, express them or manage them adequately.

When an individual suppresses feelings, the body will express them in its own language, like postures, gestures, bioelectrical changes or functional disorders. We can perceive an illness as a warning sign if we see it as a friend: a symptom can become a message to which we perhaps turned a deaf ear. It is like the last formal notice before the bailiff comes to seize what is left of our health.

Withholding one's emotions has repercussions on our respiration because it causes the diaphragm to harden. Tietze refers to the works of Wilhelm Reich, the father of bioenergy who points out that, "The reason why resistances prevent the diaphragm from moving freely is clear: the body defends itself against perceptions of pleasure or anxiety that inevitably occur during the movements of the diaphragm." A chronic hardening of the diaphragm area suggests that the patient is fighting back a rage caused by the constant repression of his or her emotions. It is not a rare occurrence to find a forward curvature of the part of the spinal column located behind the diaphragm.

On the other hand, we can also be trapped with anger. If getting angry is not bad in itself, and sometimes could be well justified, it is important to not be a too long victim of it. Out of deep breathing or counting to reduce anger, one way is to express the words coming with anger by signing them. That would surely make you laugh pretty soon. Some people torture themselves with being mad about things over which they have little control, and it eats them up inside[58]. One of my tips is to write a poem about the subject or the person I am mad about. It is made on a controlled environment; it makes me think profoundly to the problem and to find a way to express it properly or in a funny way. It is always a pleasure to read it afterward. By this, I try to make a delight of my madness! However, often it takes me time before being able to write on a tough subject, but I feel much better about it after my poems "trapped my feelings" instead of me.

Interpretation of the symptoms

According to Tietze, anxiety and sadness build up in the abdomen. The stomach especially reacts to two kinds of strong emotions: the pressing but unfulfilled desire to receive support, help and attention, and the repression of anger.

Patients who suffer from stomach ulcers appear to have a great need to be loved and cared for (patients suffering from *helicobacter pylori* can probably be excluded from this list). From a structural viewpoint, the purpose of these patients' search for human kindness is apparently to relive situations which occurred very early in life when a baby is fed, mothered and given constant attention. Psychosomatic specialists call this oral fixation.

The patient wishes to become a child again and to be fed with tenderness and love. If he or she does not succeed in driving back this desire, a conflict ensues. Since we obviously cannot, as adults, identify with

---

[58]   IBS for Dummies, p. 318-319.

this desire, we may feel ashamed because of it. This, naturally, is not felt consciously but the problem remains, and this conflict finds its expression through the body. The desire to be "fed lovingly" can manifest itself through an overproduction of gastric juices.

Psychological research suggests that children who feel rejected even in their mother's womb are constantly hungry because of permanent hyper-secretion, which their mother either cannot or does not want to release them from – unconsciously. She may suffer neurosis and, because of it, will not acknowledge that she refuses to love her child as he or she deserves. She may feel guilty and make up for it by over-feeding him. But her disappointment increases when she sees that the child remains as hungry as ever.

The intestine is extremely sensitive to emotions. In times of assimilation, upset and anger the intestine is strongly irrigated and seized by compulsive movements; the secretion then increases suddenly, irritating and ulcerating the intestinal wall.

The author considers that people suffering from intestinal ulcers are often dependent on their mothers, perfectionists, creatures of habit, and distrustful of their fellows. They are often dominated by one parent whom they fear while the other parent is more laid back and submissive. An ulcer sufferer tries to maintain balance in the family by being uncommunicative and unpredictable. They give up easily and feel overwhelmed by the most trivial events, thinking that they have to fight constantly with the energy of despair to survive. When is my ulcer due?

On the other hand, a child can be constipated when being toilet trained, a time when children are engaged in a power struggle with their mother. By holding on to their stools they may express a refusal of what they feel is a hostile environment. Such stubbornness is a symbolic act of provocation, often a source of constipation problems in adults.

Diarrhoea problems tend to symbolize an inability to face unpleasant issues. People who suffer from this are described as having an unstable disposition, as dependent, under constant tension, generally weak, demoralized and infantile.

Those who suffer from urinary retention appear to be psycho-sexually underdeveloped. They appear to respond to the demands of their urges at an infantile level, the body not distinguishing between the elimination and the genital functions. Urinary retention suggests an inability to resolve deep-seated conflicts and to let them go as an adult would.

Introspective work on the symbolism of symptoms can reveal structural emotional aspects. Finding our own symbolization is a considerable task but it can help us forgive ourselves, take care of ourselves (symptoms are merciless in expressing internal conflicts), become more active, with the ability to let go and to work at achieving more well-being. In my opinion this step could be eased with the help of professionals, whether psychologists, psychoanalysts, etc.

Depression [59]

According to Health Canada, nearly 20% of Canadians will suffer from a mental illness during their lifetime and the remaining 80% will have a family member, a friend or a colleague who suffers from this disease. Although, Muriel Schiffman, in her book "Self Therapy: Techniques for Personal Growth, Self Therapy Press" shows a good example of someone succeeding in caring oneself for her mental illness problems.

IBS can often cause or accompany a state of depression. As we saw earlier, some antidepressants reduce abdominal pain. The "Chaire en gestion de la santé et de la sécurité du travail" of Laval University has published manuals on psychological health in the workplace. They indicate that people can experience muscle tension and gastrointestinal

---

[59] *Chaire en gestion de la santé et de la sécurité du travail dans les organisations : série La santé psychologique au travail... de la définition du problème aux solutions :*
Fascicule 1 : L'ampleur du problème – L'expression du stress au travail.
Fascicule 2 : Les causes du problème – Les sources de stress au travail.
Fascicule 3 : Faire cesser le problème – La prévention du stress au travail.
Offer in : http://cgsst.fsa.ulaval.ca

disorders when they feel unable to deal with a given situation. Excessive stress levels can have physical, psychological and behavioural effects.

Tableau V Reactions related to stress		
Physical	**Psychological**	**Behavioural**
• Migraine	• Depressive mood	• Absenteeism
• Sleeping disorders	• Despair	• Drug addiction
• Muscle tension	• Boredom	• Sexual problems
• Weight problem	• Anxiety	• Impatience and
• **Gastrointestinal**	• Memory loss	aggressiveness
disorder	• Dissatisfaction	• **Dietary problems**
• High blood	• Frustration	• Drop in creativity
pressure	• Irritability	and initiative
• Allergies	• Discouragement	• Interpersonal
• High cholesterol	• Pessimism	relationship
level		problems
• Dermatological		• Inability to
ailments		tolerate frustration
		• Loss of interest
		• Isolation

Unipolar and bipolar disorders

Your doctor can determine whether your depressive feeling has developed into a mood disorder. Mood disorders can fall into the unipolar or bipolar disorder category. Unipolar depression is characterized by an almost constant depressive mood, a feeling of sadness with a lack of interest or pleasure in regular activities. Almost

Louis-Guy Lemieux, *Le Soleil, Section Santé*, January 23rd 2005, page A 10. Dawn Burstall, R. D., T. Michael Vallis, Ph. D. and Geoffrey K. Turnbull, M. D., *I.B.S. Relief, A doctor, a Dietitian and a Psychologist Provide a Team Approach to Managing Irritable Bowel Syndrome*, Chronimed Publishing, Minneapolis, 176 p.

every day for at least two weeks, a person may experience a drop in energy, sleep, appetite and concentration, become excessively worried, ambivalent, and had feelings of guilt or despair, or suicidal thoughts. At this point it is essential to consult.

Signs of bipolar disorder include depressive periods (melancholy) alternating with bouts of mania (euphoria and overexcitement). It is estimated that only 30% of the cases are diagnosed. During the manic phase there may be exaggerated feelings of well-being, energy and confidence that may be associated with increased self-esteem, reduced sleeping needs, a desire to speak constantly and irritability. Stress can trigger either a bout of depression or mania. Activity is increased but at a level that can be detrimental to the individual or to others. Until I began doing the gas evacuation exercises in my mid-thirties, I suffered from acute indigestion with passing out at the end of a period when I had felt that "everything was going especially well and under my control."

There is no cure for bipolar disorder but it can be treated successfully.

Anxiety disorder

Anxiety, or the unpleasant anticipation of a non-existent danger or threat, is a problem when it becomes excessive, persistent or uncontrollable. We know that the anxiety disorder is generalized when it is prejudicial to life in the workplace, at home or in a social environment. A diagnosis is made when, during a six-month period, a person is agitated, tired, irritable, feels dizzy, experiences chest pains, muscle cramps, palpitations, loss of concentration and sleep, and thoughts about death.

Panic disorder occurs when we fear or feel intense, painful discomfort associated with palpitations, hot flashes, shivering, a feeling of suffocation or of imminent passing out. With panic disorder the attacks come up repeatedly or without warning. With my exercises I am able to provoke the physical symptoms I experienced during panic attacks. This way I manage to release a great deal of the nervous tension.

Several studies have shown that success in life is related more to people's emotional intelligence than to their IQ. Dr Servan-Schreiber refers to the work of scientists from Yale and from New Hampshire, who define a person's emotional IQ based on their ability to:

1. Identify their emotional state and that of other people;
2. Understand the natural development of emotions;
3. Reason about their own emotions and those of other people;
4. Manage their emotions and those of other people.

These abilities are at the centre of self-control and success in society. They are the foundation of self-knowledge, self-restraint, compassion, co-operation and ability to resolve conflicts. According to Dr Damasio, our emotions are the conscious experience of a wide range of physiological reactions that control and continuously adjust the body's biological systems to the imperatives of inner and outer environments. Thus, the emotional brain is thought to have a closer relationship with the body than with the cognitive brain. A healthy open-minded attitude and the ability to manage our emotions are likely to have a favourable impact on our biological system.

It is important to develop the ability to distinguish between the occasional "blues" related to events in our lives or to IBS-related symptoms, and unipolar or bipolar depression characterized by excess. At this point it is vital to consult a health care professional.

According to the authors of the book *IBS Relief* (p. 106), we should learn to restructure our thoughts. This involves learning to assess events more positively. To do so we must avoid the following traps:

TABLE VI	
FORMATION OF NEGATIVE THOUGHTS	**DEFINITION**
Creating catastrophic scenarios	Expecting the worst. Often using the phrase, "Yes, but if…" when talking.
Fuelling thoughts that involve dichotomy (everything is black or white)	Seeing everything as totally good or totally bad, with little nuance or options.
Increasing/ minimizing emotions, events	Exaggerating negative events and minimizing the positive.
Having selective attention	Focusing only on the negative and stressful aspects of a situation and ignoring the rest.
Believing oneself to be at the centre of everything (*personalizing*)	Telling oneself that unfortunate events are caused by an element of one's character rather than hazard and circumstance.

Taking care of these aspects allows us to feel every day a little bit more comfortable, especially with ourselves. The goal here is to give us enough space to take a better care of oneself. If I do feel better, I will be able to practice more of the air evacuation exercises or breathing and relaxation techniques. By doing so, I do improve daily my emotional and physical states.

E) – OTHER EXERCICES

Researchers[60] found that a group of people who suffered from symptoms of IBS experienced a decrease in constipation, abdominal pain and gas after they began a running program. Exercise

---

[60] IBS for Dummies, p. 205.

stimulates the lymph system avoiding swollen ankles, cellulite and inflammation. Even using a mini-trampoline can provide the same benefits of regular exercise and stimulate the lymph circulation[61]. Here is some other type of exercise found in the literature.

- **Respiratory gymnastics** [62]

Respiration is the only vital function that can be controlled both by and without conscious intervention. According to Pierre Pallardy, osteopath, dietician and author, it is our duty to make the most of these possibilities. There are schools that teach respiratory therapy, to say nothing of oriental and Chinese relaxation methods which use it extensively. This underscores the importance of deep breathing.

Greti Sägesser was among the first to propose respiratory gymnastics courses in Switzerland. "Respiratory therapy helps patients with psychosomatic disorders. When respiratory energy comes back", she says, "and a person can restore contact with their own self through breathing, then they are ready to manage their problems." In his book *Les tremblements intérieurs* (p. 70), Dr Dufour maintains that deep breathing compels us to stop thinking and brings us back into the present, because we are breathing NOW!

A good respiratory rhythm stimulates people who suffer from nervous disorders, fatigue and lack of initiative. Quite the opposite, with people who are hyperactive, stressed out or tense, respiratory energy must be toned down since the ideal state is eutonia, or a

---

[61] Ibid. p. 207.
[62] Dawn Burstall, R. D., T. Michael Vallis, Ph. D., et Geoffrey K. Turnbull, M. D., *I.B.S. Relief, A doctor, a Dietitian and a Psychologist Provide a Team Approach to Managing Irritable Bowel Syndrome,* Chronimed Publishing, Minneapolis, 176 p.
Article of Thérèse Rubin in *Édicom* :
http://www.edicom.ch/sante/conseils/altern/gymresp.html
Pierre Pallardy, *Et si ça venait du ventre? Fatigue, prise de poids, cellulite, troubles sexuels, problèmes esthétiques, dépression, insomnie, mal de dos,* Robert Laffont, Paris, 2002, 257 p.

harmonious tension level. When they attain this level for the first time, respiratory gymnastics participants experience it as something unique they will try to reconnect with. Eventually, eutonia can be recaptured in a self-sufficient manner. Out of this state, for example, an active sympathetic nervous system is linked with diarrhoea.

Klara Wolf is the founder of the Swiss school of respiratory gymnastics in Brugg. Her method is based on exercises focusing on prevention, and health maintenance and recovery. The proposed exercises are suitable for all ages. To be authorized to teach respiratory gymnastics the prerequisite is a three-year study course at the Wolf School.

According to Pierre Pallardy, learning abdominal breathing is crucial to re-establishing communication between the second brain (digestive system) and the first brain. He has been teaching his technique for almost thirty years. He recommends performing respiratory exercises approximately five times within an hour, several times a day.

In the United States, a collective has closely studied various techniques for the treatment of the IBS syndrome. The authors' clinical experience supports the claim that 99% of people suffering from IBS have a thoracic or superficial respiration. People who breathe deeply and calmly use their lungs more effectively and therefore lower their respiratory rhythm, heartbeat rate and blood pressure.

How to do the exercises

To breathe deeply you have to relax the abdomen and solicit the abdominal muscles. You need to breathe in while you push out the abdomen in front of you for six to seven seconds. Then you make a pause or remain at a specific level one or two seconds before breathing out for five to seven seconds, slowly expelling as much air as possible. You can also pull in your stomach to breathe out more deeply. As we will see with the technique developed by Pierre Pallardy, you can also apply pressure on the abdomen to help evacuate the air to a maximum. With my own exercise I try to keep my lungs free from air for a while and then relax as much as possible before I begin breathing in again.

Thoracic breathing allows people with IBS to ignore their abdominal pain. They should expect, therefore, to feel some pain when they try out deep breathing. It takes time to master the technique, not being afraid of the anticipated pain and to develop the habit of deep breathing. At first you should perform the exercises when you feel calm before trying them when you are stressed or before you integrate them to your daily activities.

I try not to miss an occasion to practise deep breathing. It is especially useful when associated with the evacuation exercises. Since I am rather tense I prefer to associate deep breathing with a definite slowing down of the respiratory rhythm. I can feel its relaxing effect as soon as I begin the exercise. Moreover, deep breathing constitutes a gentle massage of the digestive system. When I first started the evacuation exercises the breathing aspect did not seem very efficient to me. The reason was that my abdomen used to be too "spasmodic." With experience I have come to appreciate deep breathing more and more. Sometimes I do it without the evacuation techniques. I often realize that after only a few minutes my digestive system reactivates, stops being atonic and calms down. The movement of gas occurs much more naturally and is less painful when my abdomen is relaxed. However, I still have to think about it because the abdominal breathing has not yet become a reflex.

Finally, who can go without the more than 20,000 daily movements associated with abdominal breathing, as opposed to thoracic breathing? What medication can replace this? Abdominal breathing can make a difference between an atonic digestive system and a fluid flow coupled with improved regularity. For anyone who suffers from constipation without dyspeptic symptoms, I recommend deep breathing to unblock the large intestine. Once you have intake air and push your abdomen muscles outward, you can gently push your intestines downward for a second or two and then relax and start breathing out. This simulates the defecation process. After few repetitions, I will often feel a gas or even a need to defecate even if I am constipated at that time. For those with dyspeptic symptoms, deep breathing must be associated with burping exercise to do the same.

- **Pierre Pallardy's approach** [63]

Pierre Pallardy, osteopath and author, maintains that by learning to take care of our abdomen and to harmonize it with the brain, we can cure all our functional disorders. For example, he surprises new patients who come to him complaining of back pain by first treating their abdomen. Most of the time he finds their abdomen is hard, spasmodic and bloated. In addition to caring for the patient he suggests that they practise a number of exercises that all start with the abdominal breathing.

According to Pierre Pallardy, respiratory exercises differ depending on whether a person hyperventilates (as in my case), or breathes superficially. In the first case the deep breathing is slow and reduces the air intake, in the other case it is more rapid. He suggests that patients perform abdominal breathing exercises a few times every hour, and more intensely once or twice a day. Although it is not easy for me to maintain this pace, I share his enthusiasm for the increased well-being it provides.

Pierre Pallardy's abdominal breathing technique is similar to mine in every way. What is specific to his is the abdominal pressure applied with the fists, or the fact of pushing down to the limit to help evacuate the air, and the intestinal massage. According to Pallardy, abdominal breathing helps the air penetrate into the abdomen. The patient's main task is then to release, unblock the diaphragm allowing the air to move freely in and out of the stomach. Even with experience I still can't tell when I swallow air. Although I have learned to chew[64]

---

[63]   Pierre Pallardy, *Et si ça venait du ventre? Fatigue, prise de poids, cellulite, troubles sexuels, problèmes esthétiques, dépression, insomnie, mal de dos*, Robert Laffont, Paris, 2002, 257 p.

[64]   Shewing properly means to chew at least 30 times by food intake. « You

my food properly, and to limit air intake while eating, I still need to belch to release it. I do suppose that the air in my stomach is more due to dyspepsia and the slow digestive process that goes with it than by air intake. In his book Pierre Pallardy does not refer to belching as a way to release the air from the abdomen.

In addition to respiration techniques Pierre Pallardy shows his patients how to massage the abdomen to relieve fatigue and release deeply buried pain. He writes: "I usually lay down on my back (or remain seated) and, instead of giving myself a gentle massage I proceed to literally crush my abdomen after pinching the skin hard causing violent pain for five or six minutes. I act with a degree of violence but I feel fine, as if this pain got the better of the deeply buried pain... these deep-seated self-massages are hard on the hands. To relax them I have to breathe deeply and regularly. I then discover the extraordinary effectiveness of this massage-respiration combination: as my fatigue drops spectacularly I get better sleep, my irritability tapers off and my abdominal pain is less and less frequent!" (p. 27-28).

When I read these lines I realized that it concerned exterior massages to help relax the abdomen, and that it produced the same results as the techniques I use, working from the inside. Although the gas evacuation exercise is not as violent, it does help bring to the surface deep-seated pain I cannot leave behind because it belongs to my childhood and is now part of my personality. Eliminating the pain caused by the gas trapped in the pit of the stomach means letting go of my status as a victim of inadequate care, and of the chief amusement of my early childhood of which I still keep a trace, not to mention the attitude. For his part Pierre Pallardy mainly suffered from hunger during childhood, which helps explain his rage.

Pierre Pallardy's method relies on seven bases: abdominal breathing, slow regular eating habits, a good diet, pleasure-sport, the dual-brain gymnastics, self-massages and abdominal meditation.

---

can accomplish almost one-third of tour digestion in your mouth. » IBS for Dummies, p. 45.

Food must be eaten regularly without stress, sitting down and in a calm setting, with a healthy appetite and above all, with pleasure. Pierre Pallardy recommends that his patients keep a diary covering these aspects, and note the composition of their meals and of the beverages they drink. He recommends a vegetarian diet (without however considering it as a cure-all), avoiding extreme diets and overeating (especially beverages, but without excluding them) and the excessive use of supplements such as antioxidants.

With regard to the sport-pleasure duet, 45 minutes endurance fast-paced walk every day is a minimum. According to other studies, you need at least twenty minutes of fast-paced walk three times a week to get a positive effect on the emotional brain. Another option is to ride a bike or practise a sport that is relatively demanding. Pallardy notes that, "No functional abdominal disorder such as constipation, bloating, painful periods, etc., can resist regular endurance sports activity." (p. 111) He refers to a Duke University study which concludes that regular sports activities practised over a period of four months have the same effect as antidepressants (Zoloft) in some patients, and that the relapse rate was clearly lower in active patients. In my case I bicycle to work (and sometimes cross country skiing in winter) all year long on an eight-kilometre course including a steep hill. All for health reasons and "combine spirit": sport, deep breathing, pleasure and useful transportation! On bad weather or to avoid too much exercising, I take the bus. But as I commute, I practice deep breathing and silent burping all along the way. I end up in a good shape and attitude at work in the morning and at home in evening. This worth at least an hour and a half exercising during the night, so that leave more time for deep sleeping.

The dual-brain gymnastics involves five exercises. But first, whatever the circumstance, he suggests that we perform the following exercise: standing up or sitting down, with the back straight, breathe in for seven to ten seconds opening up your chest as much as possible while maintaining the elbows close to the body and the fists clenched. When you breathe out, make a round back, drop your head keeping your chin flexible and digging in your hands to help pull in the abdomen to the limit.

To maintain a balance between the two brains, each movement must first be imagined, then generated and controlled by way of the abdomen in a slow, deep, continuous manner synchronized with abdominal breathing. All the exercises must be performed about five times in a row at first (more in the case of athletes) and, when you get into the habit you can perform two or three series of these five exercises:

- Standing with legs apart, knees bent and arms stretched out, back slightly rounded out, imagine yourself pulling a load towards you for seven to ten seconds while breathing in. When your fists are close to your waist you can pause, open the palm of your hands and push your imaginary load in front of you while breathing out. Make a round back, let your head fall between your arms and pull in your abdomen as much as you can;
- On all fours on the floor, picture yourself pushing a load while expanding your abdomen. As you breathe out, imagine that the abdomen is pulling the load in. Make a round back as much as possible;
- While lying on your back, breathe as you inflate your abdomen and do some pull-ups (head and arms only) while breathing out and drawing in your abdomen as much as possible;
- On your back, hands behind the chin, legs bent, put one of your ankles over one knee while you breathe in and touch your other knee with your elbow. After doing this a few times, repeat the exercise with your other elbow and knee;
- Standing with arms alongside the body, clench your fists while breathing in and open your hands while breathing out.

To give yourself a soothing massage you need to lightly touch your abdomen without applying any pressure, alternating clockwise and counterclockwise circles. Then, with both hands on the abdomen, apply pressure as you expand the abdomen and breathe in, squashing it while breathing out. Then, with your hands, apply a vibrating motion to your abdomen. Finally, keeping the palm of your hand in contact with the abdomen, knead the skin and conjunctive tissue for one minute. Pierre Pallardy also recommends what he refers to as "self-massage treatments", consisting of pressure applied on specific points (meridians). Another possibility is to knead even more thoroughly. Finally, to get rid of the cellulitic infiltration you have to pinch and roll (grabbing the skin between thumb and fingers with both hands and rolling it between your fingers). These exercises are described more thoroughly in his book.

Abdominal meditation consists of laying your open palms on your belly as you try to feel the flux of internal fluids. Picture the flow of the gastric meatus as a sinewy river encountering various obstacles. You must focus on the painful points (the obstacles) or the skin close to these points to get these areas to relax. You can also move your hands slowly from the sternum to the groin. This meditation can help revive painful memories. Pallardy mentions that you need to practice for several months, ten minutes at a time twice a day, before you can feel the abdomen coming alive beneath your hands.

• EMDR [65]

In his book *Guérir le stress, l'anxiété et la dépression sans médicaments ni psychanalyse*, Dr David Servan-Schreiber deals at length with neuroemotional integration through eye movements (the acronym EMDR is short for *Eye Movement Desensitization and Reprocessing*). This technique seems very effective in treating the neuropsychological aspects of post-traumatic stress disorder (PTSD). Dr Servan-Schreiber refers to research conducted by Dr Stéphane LeDoux showing that fear is not learned by way of the neocortex but rather goes directly

---

[65]   David Servan-Schreiber, M. D. and psychiatrist, *Guérir le stress, l'anxiété et la dépression sans médicaments ni psychanalyse*, Robert Laffont, Paris, 2003, 302 p.

to the emotional brain, which never unlearns it. The emotional scars of our limbic brain are apparently ready to resurface as soon as the vigilance of our cognitive brain and its control capacity weakens. According to the EMDR theory, the trauma related information is blocked in the nervous system where it is recorded in its original form. This network, rooted in the emotional brain and disconnected from rational knowledge, becomes a bundle of undigested, dysfunctional information which the slightest reminder can reactivate.

No other technique has been researched as much and within so short a time in order to test its effectiveness. Many hesitate to adopt it, however it is increasingly considered to be as effective as the best, most easily tolerated and quickest existing treatments. Today it is officially recognized as a means of treating PTSD by, among others, the American Psychological Association, the International Society for Traumatic Stress Study and the United Kingdom Health Department.

The technique consists in recalling the traumatic memory in all its visual, emotional, cognitive and physical components. The therapist then asks the patient to follow his rapid hand motions from left to right to induce eye movements such as those experienced during heavy sleep. This stimulates the adaptive information treatment system we all possess. Once stimulated, this system digests the dysfunctional imprint.

Although painful at first, because it brings back memories that may be recorded in the entire body, alternating rest and brief stimulation periods helps patients quickly pass through all the stages of healing of post-traumatic shock (anxiety, fear, anger, rationalization, compassion). Even if the trauma occurred in childhood, this link to adulthood helps eliminate the feelings of powerlessness and submissiveness associated with past dangers. Patients rapidly become functional as if they had finally cured their deep emotional scars. However, EMDR is apparently not as effective in treating the symptoms not related to past trauma, or biological depressions, psychoses or dementia.

- **Heart coherence** [66]

For doctors the great variation in heart rate resulting from an effort, for example, is a sign of good health. Moreover, heart rate can be dissociated from the brain: do we not sometimes refer to arrhythmia? An approach created by the Institute of HearthMath in California involves several stages promoting the achievement of heart coherence. According to Dr Servan-Schreiber, once heart coherence has been established, the patients realize that they possess an intuitive inner self that has guided them all their lives. They develop also compassion for this inner self.

To establish contact between heart and brain, we must first turn our attention to ourselves. Deep breathing exercises can help. As Dr Servan-Schreiber tells us, "The revolution, i.e., inner peace – is [...] at the end of the exhalation [...]." After approximately fifteen seconds of stabilization, the focus must be directed towards the heart region, as if allowing you to breathe through it and feel it becoming lighter as a result of this ventilation. The third stage consists in *connecting* with the sensation of heat and the expansion coming from the heart. Dr Servan-Shreiber tells us that our heart is especially sensitive to gratefulness, gratitude and love. We will often feel a smile gently forming on our lips. This is a sign that coherence has been established. You can then question your heart. If, to a question you ask yourself the warmth reappears this indicates that you can progress along the proposed path, if not, you should avoid it. You can thus find avenues to bring together the heart and the brain.

After going through a difficult period in 2003 and 2004, I had to drop several activities so that I could focus on my work and family. Despite my efforts I felt I had reached what I call a "depressive feeling", which I could not get rid of in 2005. Since the heart coherence exercise is perfectly in tune with my relaxation technique I got into the habit of practising it, especially when I got up in the morning. This exercise let me feel that it is going to be a great day and

---

[66] Ibid.

that everything will be all right, whatever the tribulations or pain I may encounter during that day. This is the exercise I found most successful in helping me get rid of this depressive feeling. Moreover, I feel a notable improvement of my energy and concentration capability. A great aspect of this technique is that it made me have a slight control over my optimistic attitude. This way I can become more optimistic while I judge that could be good to me.

I am thinking of developing the heart coherence exercise by combining it with the good working order of the entire digestive system… so that everything may "be all right!" It should be recalled that formerly, such expressions as "How are you?" and "Are you going well?" used to refer to intestinal functions. To parody Dr Devroede, I would like to refer to a fundamental ("fond-amental") coherence exercise. I find that the heart coherence exercise helps me forget about possible intestinal pain that could come up during the day. While I don't sleep early in the morning, I do practice that fundamental coherence exercise. It is for me as if I push relaxation (decontraction of the abdominal zone) as much as I can. For few months since the end of 2010, I do practice this internal exercise. I then feel a deep sweetness and pleasure in my abdomen for minutes and repeat it many times before getting up. This gives me much more inner space to tolerate everyday's stress.

F) – WHAT SHOULD WE TAKE

• **Time**

One important factor to alleviate IBS symptoms is giving us time. We must take our time to know us better, to try exercise, diet and to live our ordinary life with less stress. The book IBS for Dummies (p. 255) mentions to wake up half an hour than usual to give us time to work up to morning symptoms and relax up to work.

The adaptation for my new job was so difficult in 2010 that I stopped for almost a year to work on this book. Since I wanted to give me more time, let say quality time, I started to work back on it because that's a place where I do what I want. For me, even though it is not a paying job, it is one which I found "adaptation" much easier. I must than thank you, readers, to be a reason to giving myself such a time toward a partly happier life at work! It is for me an example of what I call a humane process, like IBS, to part from the worst and working out up for the better.

Speaking of time, the book IBS for Dummies says that timing is everything when comes the time to talk about your problems especially at work. "...you may want to consider having a discussion with your boss about your illness. Together, you may be able to come up with ways that you can keep your IBS from interfering with your productivity and comfort at work... If you can muster the courage to tell the truth you may find that you get a lot of support – perhaps even from people who have personal experience with what you're going through.[67]"

Your boss must know that your condition may make it difficult to be on time for work, that you need to be close to a bathroom, that you may have to rush out of a meeting suddenly, that you may have to stay at home sometimes. That will allow you to know what kind of a boss you have and, at least, will help you feel less troubled at "times". The book IBS for Dummies gives other tips to regain power in the workplace like focus on what you can control; be as public as you need to be and as private as you want to be; reach beyond relief, go for the satisfaction; control your message (to whom, when, how).

• Medication[68]

In general, drugs therapies for IBS consist of laxatives for constipation, bulking agents for diarrhoea, antispasmodics for pain, and antidepressants for stress. A survey conducted by the International Foundation for Functional Gastrointestinal Disorders showed that only one-third of people surveyed reported that they were satisfied with the results.

---

[67] IBS for Dummies, p. 257.
[68] Ibid. pp. 146-147.

• The placebo [69]

Placebos are make-believe treatments or medicines that do not contain any active ingredients, but whose psychological effectiveness can reduce the intensity of most pain by 30% to 60%. For centuries there has been a controversy as to whether the placebo is either an unacceptable hoax or an invaluable blessing. What we call a "placebo" is any medical act giving a subject the illusion of a medically approved therapy (M. Yvonneau, 1962). The placebo effect is the difference between the observed change and the change imputable to the active elements of a medication (P. Pichot, 1961). In this regard, doctors learn that the placebo effect cannot be discounted, even when an active medication is prescribed.

Already in Montaigne's era, a medical doctor had written that his presence was in itself sufficient to cure many human beings. Petr Skrabanek and James McCormick, both professors at Dublin University, remind us that an 1890 judgment confirmed that British law did not favour placebos. The legality of its benefits had had its day. The authors add that the doctor's belief in the effectiveness of his treatment and the patient's trust in the doctor work in synergy. The remedy then guarantees an improvement, sometimes a cure.

According to A. Hrobjartsson and others, (New England Journal of Medicine 2001; 344 : 1594-602) the placebo brings a subjective or objective improvement in 30% to 40% of patients in varying clinical

---

[69] P. Kissel et D. Barrucand, *Placebos et effet placebo en médecine*, Masson, Paris, 1964.
Articles in *Agora* : http://www.agora.fr
P. Skrabaneck et J. McCormick, *Idées folles, idées fausses en médecine*, Odile Jacob ed. Coll. Opus, Paris, 1997, 196 p.
Articles in E-santé : http://www.e-sante.fr
M. de Montaigne, *Essais, tome I, Livre premier*, chap. XXI, *Le livre de poche. Librairie générale française, Paris,* 1972, in B. Lachaux and P. Lemoine, *Placebo, un médicament qui cherche la vérité*, Medsi/McGraw-Hill, Paris, 1988.
W. Grant Thompson, M. D., Gut Reactions – Topics in Functional Gastrointestinal Disease: What are Placebos? Are they good for you?, *Participate,* vol. 11, n° 4, Winter 2002, IFFGD, http://www.iffgd.org

situations such as those involving pain, asthma, hypertension, even a heart attack. However, by going over more than 114 studies on pain, the authors conclude that the placebo does not have a direct effect and acts moderately, but not significantly, on chronic subjective symptoms. However, it is generally recognized as significant in the case of people with FDDs. Moreover, other studies have shown that, in circumstances, a lactose tablet can relieve not only the patients' anxiety but also his or her pain, nausea, vomiting, palpitation, shortness of breath, or other symptoms. Patients expect relief when they get a medication, and sometimes they obtain relief by the very fact of expecting it.

R. de la Fuente Fernandez and others (Science 2001; 293) refer to a survey conducted with six Parkinson patients who, upon functional imaging, responded as effectively to the placebo as to medication in respect of dopamine released. In each of these Parkinson patients the placebo seemed all the more active when the waiting and the hope were great, which is consistent with the classical data. The placebo therefore seems to be one of the best natural medicine prototypes.

Because of the placebo effect, scientists only recognize the effectiveness of a medication after a double-blind random study is conducted using a placebo. This type of study helps isolate the therapeutic effect of a new medication and match the appropriate medication to a patient's specific condition. In the case of FDDs, the patient's variable condition can also bring on improvement naturally during the course of treatment, irrespective of the placebo effect or the active components of a medication.

Although there are few studies on the placebo effect, it has been observed that a placebo injection is more effective than a placebo (medication), that a large pill is more effective than a small one, and that the colour of the pill is important. When administered by a physician a medication gives better results than when administered by a nurse, a mail-ordered product is not as effective, and the pain is relieved quicker if the medication is followed by a placebo. Moreover, everyone reacts differently to a placebo.

There is also the nocebo effect, the opposite of the placebo effect, which occurs when a patient's condition deteriorates after the doctor's visit. "See the doctor and die!" my father would say. This effect can also be observed in patients who have just been diagnosed, or who have just taken their medicine. There is also the "voodoo effect" where the physician is seen as a bad witch-doctor or, in other societies, as the medicine man who can call out to bad spirits. For example, a study has revealed doctors' ineffectiveness when they see IBS patients who are secretly afraid of having cancer. What appears to be the key factor here is the relationship between patient and doctor. From this perspective, the good doctor is actually a placebo.

The placebo effect also extends to the apparatus and techniques used by chiropractors, naturopaths and other non-medical practitioners who use heat, hydrotherapy, manipulation, massages, light, etc. In conjunction with a physiological effect, they create a psychological impact enhanced by the patient-practitioner relationship.

Dr Barry Beyerstein, psychologist, emphasizes that there are physical as well as psychological aspects in pain. Successful quacks and healers rely on faith; they have highly charismatic personalities enabling them to influence the psychological variables that modulate pain in gullible people. According to Dr Stephen Barrett, editor of Quackwatch.com, people who turn to placebos do not usually draw any beneficial effect from them, and their use is basically a rip-off.

So, what kind of attitude should we have towards the effects or the use of placebos? Their scientific authority is undeniable since studies which fail to take them into account are considered unscientific. As for the rest, Aristotle is the one who answers my questions, the philosopher for whom "is good what is suitable;" and the greatest value is friendship. So why not seek our doctor's friendship?

Homeopathy [70]

Dr Stephen Barrett gives a detailed account of homeopathy on his Web site. The following is a summary of his thoughts. He believes homeopathy is one of the greatest existing hoaxes. Homeopathic "remedies" enjoy a unique status in the health market. They are authorized under the 1938 United States Federal Food, Drug, and Cosmetic Act recognizing as medicines all the substances included in the United States' Homeopathic Pharmacopoeia. However, these products are not subject to the same criteria as other medicines. Therefore, the Food and Drug Administration does not guarantee their effects. Yet, many insurance companies cover homeopathic products, and some public health insurance systems, as in France, even recognize them and partly refund their costs.

Based on mistaken beliefs

The origin of homeopathy dates back to the late 1700s, when Samuel Hahnemann (1755-1843), a German physician, began formulating its basic principles. He partly based his theory on the law of infinitesimal, which maintains that the less an ingredient is contained in a given substance the more active it is. This is the opposite of what has always been demonstrated by the pharmacological science. Thus, the effectiveness, as the ineffectiveness, of homeopathic products is relatively unprovable.

The conclusions of the Homeopathic Pharmacopoeia are not the result of scientific assessment but of trials conducted at the end of the 1800s and early 1900s. The fact that homeopathic remedies were

---

[70] http://www.allerg.qc.ca/homeopathie.html
http://www.passeportsante.net/fr/actualites/nouvelles/fiche.aspx?doc=2005082705
http://www.passeportsante.net/fr/therapies/guide/fiche.aspx?doc=homeopathie_th
A. Shang, K. Huwiler-Muntener and others, *Are the clinical effects of homoeopathy placebo effects? Comparative study of placebo-controlled trials of homoeopathy and allopathy. Lancet* 2005, August-Septembre; 366 (9487) : 726-32.

not as dangerous as the remedies proposed by the 1900 century medical orthodoxy encouraged their use. The last genuine school of homeopathy closed in the United States in the late 1920s.

Homeopathic remedies are prescribed according to the patient's "constitutional type". There is for example, the Ignatia type, a nervous individual who cries a lot and can't stand cigarette smoke; the Pulsatilla type, which suites as young fair haired, blue eyed women, friendly but shy. The Nux Vomica type is considered to be aggressive, rough, ambitious and hyperactive. The Sulphur type is independent, etc.

Remedies that are basically placebos

Soluble homeopathic products are diluted into 9 or 99 parts of water; the insoluble products are crushed and pulverized in similar proportions, with powdered lactose (milk sugar). Part of the diluted remedy is then diluted even more, and the process in repeated until the desired concentration is obtained. The 1 per 10 dilutions are designated by the Roman number X 1X = 1/10, 3X = 1/1 000, 6X = 1/1 000 000). In the same way, 1 per 100 dilutions are designated by the Roman number C (1C = 1/100, 3C = 1/1 000 000, and so on). Today, most remedies range between 6X and 30X, but 30C products or more are available. The 30X dilutions indicate that the original substance has been diluted 1 000 000 000 000 000 000 000 000 000 000 times.

For example, Dr Robert L. Park, managing director of the American Physical Society, notes that if the smallest quantity of a substance is a molecule, a 30C solution would have at least one molecule of the original substance, dissolved in a container that would be thirty billion times bigger than the Earth.

The *Oscillococcinum*, a 200C product designed to relieve cold or flu symptoms, requires small amounts of a duck's liver and heart to be diluted. In a year, substances from a single duck are required to make a product whose sales amounted to twenty million dollars in 1996. Dr Park notes that to expect to have one molecule of the medicinal substance in the 30X tablets means that you would need two billion tablets, amounting to a total of approximately a thousand tons of lactose, over and above the other impurities that the lactose could contain.

In 1990, an article published in the Review of Epidemiology referred to an analysis of forty studies that compared homeopathic treatments with standard treatments, a placebo, or no treatment at all. The authors concluded that all studies except three had a faulty methodology and that only one out of three had positive results. The authors concluded that there was no evidence that homeopathic treatment was more effective than a placebo.

Another study of trials published in The Lancet in 1997 concludes that it is impossible to draw undeniable proof of the effectiveness of homeopathy for a specific medical intervention. Other studies slightly lean towards the effectiveness of homeopathy, and the collected data excludes the possibility that the placebo effect is the only cause.

In December 1996 a lengthy report was published by the Homeopathic Medicine Research Group (HMRG), a group of experts gathered together by the Commission of the European Communities. Its conclusions were that most homeopathic research is without value; no homeopathic product proved effective in treating any medical condition. The National Council Against Health Fraud warns that the sectarian nature of homeopathy raises serious questions about the credibility of those who study its effects.

According to a study by Drs A. Shang, K. Huwiler-Muntener et al., published by The Lancet in September 2005, the effects of homeopathy are similar to those of a placebo. After studying 110 clinical trials, the authors analysed those that had the better methodology. Only nine trials involving classic medicine, and 21 involving homeopathy, met these criteria. The result was that the classic treatments were superior to the placebo, but that homeopathy was not. This study had been commissioned by the Swiss Government to help make decision-making easier in the case of homeopathic medicines. The

Swiss health insurance savings banks thus no longer refund the costs of homeopathy.

According to Dr Barrett, spontaneous remission is also a factor in the popularity of homeopathy. Most people who attribute their "cure" to homeopathic products would have had the same results without them. It is his opinion that US Food and Drug Administration (FDA) officials consider homeopathy as relatively innocuous (compared, for instance, to products whose effects are still unproven and which are sold as cancer or AIDS treatments); and therefore that the pre-eminence of homeopathy can be found elsewhere.

• Phytotherapy [71]

According to Passeportsante.net, the use of medicinal plants is the most widespread form of medicine on the planet. Their popularity has resurfaced since the 1970s, especially as a result of the undesirable side-effects of synthetic medications. The World Health Organization (WHO) and the European Community established agencies whose task is to take inventory of the traditional uses of medicinal plants, validate them scientifically and gain a better understanding of their underlying mechanisms.

However, herbal medicines are often sold by naturopaths, acupuncturists, iridologists, chiropractors, unlicensed herbalists, etc. They generally prescribe them for a wide range of health problems. Some of these specialists are not actually qualified to make medical diagnoses or assess how these products compare with accepted medications. The book IBS for Dummies (p. 164) recommend the

---

[71] http://www.allerg.qc.ca/minedherb.html
http://www.passeportsante.net/fr/therapies/guide/fiche.aspx?doc=phytotherapie_th
http://www.e-sante.fr/fr/magazine_sante/autres_maladies/plantes_meilleure_digestion-9618-214-art.htm
Collection Protégez-vous et Passeportsanté.net, Guide des produits de santé naturels, 2006, Protégez-vous, Montréal, 96 p.; http://www.pv.qc.ca.

site of Heather Von Vorous who had IBS since she was 9 years old (www.helpforibs.com).

Medicinal plants enthusiasts like to stress that almost half of the medications in use today are derived from plants. However, medicinal products contain specific amounts of active ingredients. The herbs, in their natural state, can vary quite a bit from one batch to the next, and they often contain chemical products that may cause side effects.

According to Monique Lalancette and Léon René de Cotret, of Passeportsante.net, there is a trend, herbal medicine, which is centered on an empirical knowledge of plants and their historically recognized effects. It involves the effects of the plant as a whole on any individual. Most of the time, herbalists are the ones preparing the plant mixtures and their presentation (powder, capsule, crème, herbal tea, etc.). Another trend, phytotherapy, is more centered on biochemical knowledge, and focuses on the symptoms of diseases and the action of the plants' active principles. However, research and development in the field of phytotherapy are not easy to fund since the plants cannot be patented. Therefore, it is impossible to make research efforts pay off. However, thanks to better research protocols, the synergic action of the various constituents is starting to be understood better and scientifically accepted. However, according to Dr Barrett of Quackwatch, the best source of information on herbs, the Natural Medicines Comprehensive Database (http://www.naturaldatabase.com) which inventoried close to a thousand different herbs and dietary supplements has only identified 15 % of them as safe and 11 % as effective for the indications mentioned.

According to Dr Barrett of the United States, the herbs used for preventive or therapeutic purposes are subject to the drug regulation agency, which is under federal jurisdiction. To circumvent the law, these products are sold as foods or dietary supplements. Since all herbs are not subject to the same rules as regular medicines, there is no legal standard for their processing, gathering or packaging. Several studies mentioned in Quackwatch indicate that some products labelled as herbs do not contain any useful ingredients; others simply do not contain the main ingredient they advertise. When it is present, the amount indicated rarely matches the actual content.

Products that contain numerous herbal ingredients can have side effects that are difficult to predict. A 1999 survey conducted by the magazine "Prévention" reveals that 12 % of medicinal herb users report harmful effects. American law will not prohibit a product that often causes harmful side effects. The FDA instead puts out a warning.

According to Passeportsante.net, some plants are toxic, while others can be harmful to the user's health when they interact with other plants, medicines or supplements. The site indicates the potential harmful interactions of some plants.

During my "digestive career" I used a number of plant-based dietary supplements. Among those I tried there is vegetable coal, a supplement said to absorb harmful bacteria in the stomach. My impression was that it provided relief from gas for a few days, but that the intestinal flora rapidly renewed itself and the gas returned even more fiercely. I also tried digestive enzymes (papaya) but I felt that they had no more effect than a placebo. I got results with a plant supplement, Physozyme-D, intended to control acidobasic imbalance. However, I consider, in my case, grapefruit or grapefruit juice was more effective.

I also tried various "digestive" herbal teas. These preparations often contain balm (*melisa officinalis*), a perennial plant with a lemony smell. It has grown in my garden for a number of years, so I occasionally infuse a few fresh leaves during the summer. Balm should not be boiled or brewed for too long because it tends to lose its flavour. However, as with other digestive preparations, I get the feeling that their main benefit comes from drinking... the hot water they are infused in. When I was a child, a family friend from France used to tell us that: "When nothing works, a bowl of hot water makes everything to pass... by the lower or the upper channel." My other preferred herbal tea is mint, especially spearmint, which I also grow in my garden. I make them dry in summer to be able to consume them all year long. Since a few months, I prepare one of these herbal teas while starting my day at the office. It gives some warmth in my stomach helping it to relax early in the day.

Of course, I haven't tried all the supplements. However, merely reading their constitutive elements can often demystify the endless benefits mentioned in the publicity. For instance, Floralax is a supplement composed of psyllium, aloe vera and prunes. So, why not just eat fibres or fresh prunes, either raw or soaked in water? Another supplement called Bio Superaliment (BSA) consists of various dried algae, including spiruline. Since this product is rich in omega-3, why not eat the fresh algae or use omega-3 supplements, whose benefits are more widely demonstrated? I will spare you the unending, almost miraculous, so-called benefits listed in brochures dealing with this type of products.

According to an article by Étienne Genovefa, a reporter for *E-santé*, many plants contain eupectic essential oils that relieve digestive problems. These plants include caraway, dill or fennel, which also help fight aerophagy and abdominal bloating. Other plant species such as boldo stimulate the digestive functions after a heavy meal. Pineapple, which is rich in bromeline, also acts positively on digestion, as do the papaya and ginger, an aromatic tonic widely used to relieve dyspepsia. Finally, plants such as artichoke, rosemary or black radish stimulate liver functions and improve digestion.

In 2006, the magazine *Protégez-vous*, in collaboration with Passeportsante.net, published its "Guide des produits de santé naturels." If you suffer from stomach or digestive problems, the following plants are recommended: artichoke, milk-thistle, turmeric, ginger, devil's claw and bitter orange.

Artichoke relieves digestive problems and lowers blood cholesterol levels. Its active element, cynarine, has not been used as a medication since the 1980s. In Europe, milk-thistle is used in combination with medications to treat liver disorders. However, since these disorders are not easily treated, milk-thistle should be taken under a doctor's supervision. These two products are not recommended for anyone who is allergic to compounds (aster, camomile, daisy, etc.) Curcuma is a powerful antioxidant used to treat digestive problems and prevent cancer by means of its active ingredient, the curcuma. Ginger relieves nausea and vomiting during pregnancy. It prevents travel sickness, seasickness, as well as various minor digestive problems. Turmeric and ginger should not be taken in large quantities by pregnant women. Devil's claw stimulates the appetite and relieves digestive problems but it should not be taken together with anticoagulants. Bitter orange is used in Chinese medicine for a number of digestive problems. However, it has many contraindications, especially when combined with caffeine. It is said to facilitate weight loss.

• The diet

The effect of diet on an irritable colon varies from one person to the next. Dietary fats are known to be triggering factors because they slow down the gastric meatus transit. Corn, wheat and even fibre can trigger symptoms for some people. In others, adding fibre to the diet such as bran or a psyllium preparation helps regularize intestinal function. Monosodium glutamate can also cause severe irritable colon symptoms (as in my case). In general, most foods and food additives can cause irritable bowel symptoms. If so, the symptoms are easily reproduced: every time one eats the triggering substance the same symptoms appear. Keeping a diary of the symptoms and diet for at least a week helps identify the foods that trigger the reaction.

Approximately 17% of individuals are unable to digest milk or milk products. The enzyme that breaks down the lactose is absent or in a lower quantity in their digestive system. These people experience the same symptoms as those who suffer from IBS. Dairy not broken down properly by enzyme attracts a large amount of fluid in order to dilute it which results in watery diarrhoea. The treatment consists in excluding milk from the diet. Sometimes, butter can be tolerated since the part of the milk which is soluble in water has been largely removed.

During periods of overwork or exhaustion, the production of gas in the stomach and intestines can increase considerably. We may get the feeling that all the foods we eat are transformed into gas. Paying attention to what we eat can help. Thanks to the evacuation exercises, I can digest pretty much anything and, naturally, eliminate gas even though I feel there is so much of it. However, I would recommend a good diet combination, i.e., a good ratio of green and root vegetables, as well as well-balanced meals in terms of acidity. For example, the following foods should not be eaten at the same meal: pasta, white sauce, bread and cake. A pasta meal is well-balanced when it is associated with a tomato-based sauce (slightly acid), a green vegetable and fruit for dessert. However, you must avoid dessert right after a meal to avoid fermentation in the stomach.

As for dietary restrictions, the only ones I would consider are refined sugar, the foods described as gas generators, and foods that one cannot tolerate or is allergic to. With the evacuation exercises, the gas generating foods (cauliflower, broccoflower, potato chips, starchy foods, tofu, beans, soda water and fizzy drinks, etc.) are acceptable in moderation. However, researches show that dieting up to one fruit and one meat and one vegetable, for example, is effective with 66 % of patients compare with 50 % for those who would limit themselves to a few of each.

In my opinion, prohibiting alcohol and caffeine is relatively counterproductive. Taken in moderation, they are beneficial. Alcohol is a relaxant, a sought-after effect when high nervous tension accompanies the gas. As for caffeine, it is an excellent stimulant for those days when we need to do intellectual work, for example. Caffeine also helps relieve temporarily the general or built-up fatigue experienced by IBS sufferers. The benefits of a stimulant such as caffeine should not be underestimated, especially when we see how important performance is in the workplace nowadays. Coffee breaks also provide an opportunity to stop what we're doing for a few minutes and socialize. Like alcohol, however, coffee should be drunk in moderation.

As part of a therapeutic process, we can turn to some foods to obtain the desired effects. For example, I eat legumes (chickpeas, lentils, peas, beans, etc.) to stimulate gas in the large intestine when I feel I need to dream to solve a problem that can't be solved by "reason" alone. In some African tribes, healers eat lentils to heighten their visions.

IBS for Dummies suggests using coconut, flax, olive and sunflower oils for a person with IBS, since they have smaller chain fatty acids than found in polyunsaturated oils (soy, corn and other vegetables oils). Smaller chains fatty acids help rebuilt body tissue while longer chain ones are more difficult to digest leading to inflammation and irritation responses for people with intestinal problems.

Calling upon a dietician has obvious advantages. First of all, dieticians generally recommend doing a follow-up of the foods eaten so as to associate them with our health status. Although I am not really knowledgeable in that area, I heard many people tell me that they had solved their problems by following the advice of a dietician. I feel that it is very important to do a dietary follow-up. For example, flu can be the result of a salmonella infection, and it takes four days for the symptoms to appear. The same can be said about the effects of bad dietary habits, especially when a diet is too acid or too alkaline. A poor diet can increase the symptoms related to allergies or stimulate gas production. The treatment of gas problems can be made easier with a follow-up, a change of dietary habits or a better food combination if necessary.

Foods that are low gas generators

Legumes: asparagus, avocado, Swiss chard, carrots, green peas, yellow beans, mushrooms, zucchini.

Fruits: canned, peeled apple, tomato, grapes, kiwi, nectarine, citrus fruits (orange, grapefruit, lemon, clementine, etc.), peach, pear.

Meats and others: eggs, fish, red meat, olives, yogurt.

Since the discomfort caused by gas limits our food choices, we should make sure that our diet is at least complete and adequate. Among the essential nutriments we should find in our diets we find beta-carotene (or vitamin A), vitamin C and folate. Vitamins A and C are antioxidants and folate protects against diseases such as spina bifida.

The following foods are generally well tolerated by people who suffer from IBS. Select these foods, preferably cooked, as often as possible.

Table VII		
Vitamin A	Vitamin C	Folate
Carrot	Orange/orange juice	Orange/orange juice
Pumpkin	Grapefruit/grapefruit juice	Spinach or Swiss chard
Sweet potato	Tomato/tomato juice	Asparagus
Spinach or Swiss chard	Cooked potato, peel left on	
Winter squash	Spinach or Swiss chard	

If you feel better after a six-week trial, the authors of the book "I.B.S. Relief" suggest to gradually reintroducing a few foods, especially those that you miss the most.

To improve my dietary balance I often try to add legumes to my diet. Since legumes are vegetable proteins, I consider that they are less damaging to life and the environment than animal proteins, especially meat. However, as you know, gas invariable increases after I eat those foods. I have also tried Beano, which is composed of an enzyme that promotes the digestion of legumes. However, I did not experience significant improvement as a result. It is also a relatively expensive product. I would rather eat legumes in moderation when I feel relatively well.

My favourite recipes

For breakfast, here is a recipe that contains fruit for the day, and a fair amount of dietary fibre (without starchy foods or refined sugar):

For two:

Table VIII	
Ingredients	**Preparation method**
• 1 banana • 2 tablespoons (10 ml) of wheat germ (optional) • 4 tablespoons (20 ml) of wheat bran • 4 tablespoons (20 ml) of muesli • 2 tablespoons (10 ml) of 15% cream • ½ cup (120 ml) of plain yogurt (preferably biological) • 4 dates or 2 figs cut in pieces (optional) • 1 tablespoon (5 ml) of dried Sultana raisins • 1/3 cup (75 ml) of canned or fresh fruits • a few strawberries, raspberries, blueberries or blackberries whenever possible	In two soup bowls or two fairly large dessert bowls: • split the banana in half, place one half banana in each bowl and mash thoroughly with a fork • add the wheat germ, raisins, wheat bran, muesli and cream (mix well) • add yogurt, dates and canned or fresh fruits • decorate with seasonal fruits

To reduce the sugar content, remove raisins and dates. If you are oversensitive to dairy products, remove cream.

For a main course, here few recipes adapted from the "Thon à la Julie" (in a recipe book published by the *Cercles des Fermières du Québec, Tome 3*, p. 87.) which include a wide variety of nutriments. The quantities are for two people.

All the recipes contain a home-made mayonnaise base:

Table IX	
Ingredients	Preparation method
• ¼ cup (60 ml) of cold pressed extra virgin olive oil • 1 egg yolk or 1 whole egg (optional) or 2 tablespoons of lemon juice • 1 teaspoon of Dijon mustard or harissa, to taste • 1 garlic clove	Using a blender or a fork, make an emulsion by mixing all the ingredients, starting with the mustard or lemon juice and the olive oil.

Other basic ingredients:

Table X	
Ingredients	Preparation method
• ¼ cup (60 ml) of olive oil (any variety, to taste) • 1 marinated gherkin, unsweetened • 1 can of whole white tuna pepper and Provencal seasonings, Greek or Italian, to taste (above all, no salt, it's already very salty)	These ingredients can be cut in small pieces mixed with the mayonnaise or mixed in the blender.

Variations:

Table XI	
Ingredients	Preparation method
For people suffering from diarrhoea: • 1 or 2 cups of cooked brown rice	Take all the mixed ingredients, lay them over the cooled rice or mix them in. Serve immediately or refrigerate overnight (this is the basic "Tuna à la Julie").
For people suffering from constipation: • 6 whole leaves of Roman lettuce or a parsley bunch finely chopped	Take all the mixed ingredients, and place them on the leaves (three leaves per person). Looks like vegetable tacos. Another option is to cut the lettuce in pieces and mix them in a salad with the rest of the ingredients.
For people with an acidic system: • 2 slices of health bread or pasta (preferably gluten free is you are gluten sensitive)	Mix all the ingredients in the blender and spread lavishly on the bread (fresh or toasted). With pasta: heat the ingredients and serve as a sauce.
For people with an alkaline system (my case): • 1 or 2 whole tomatoes • 6 whole leaves of Roman lettuce or a bunch of parsley finely chopped.	Add the chopped or crushed tomato to the rest of the recipe in the blender. You can eat it as is, or on whole Roman lettuce leaves, or in a salad.

For me, these recipes are delicious, well-balanced, easy to digest, and tend to restore the balance of the digestive system. I recommend using them two to three times a week.

For lunch, the book IBS for Dummies (p. 192-193) suggests a salad with a healthy dressing that I use often: half a cup (120 ml) of cold pressed olive oil or coconut oil, one forth of a cup (60 ml) of lemon juice, lime juice or apple cider vinegar, two gloves of garlic and half a teaspoon (2 ml) of Dijon mustard. It also suggests for a soup to mix with a box of vegetable soup a 10 ounce package of precooked wild rice, 12 ounce can of coconut milk, a small bag of organic frozen vegetables and a teaspoon (5 ml) or more of curry powder and/or turmeric to taste.

To restore the digestive system's pH balance

To help restore an adequate acidobasic balance, we can introduce acid foods (citrus fruits, tomatoes, grapefruit juice, and vinegar) and reduce alkaline foods (starchy foods, green vegetables, legumes) for an alkaline system: do the reverse if your system is acid. For example, if your system is too acid (make sure to test the acidic level of your urine with blotting paper: heartburn does not necessarily indicate an acid system), a green vegetable soup, a serving of cheese with a slice of health bread, should help. If your system is alkaline, you should instead opt for a tomato salad with an oil and balsamic vinegar vinaigrette.

Finally, as Dr Pallardy says, eat slowly, regularly, with your mouth closed, and especially with enjoyment!

- **Dietary supplements**

Dietary fibre[72]

The recommended daily amount of dietary fibre is 20 to 35 g (more or less than 1 once). On average, people in Quebec eat half of the

---

[72] Josiane Cyr, Nutritionist, *Le Soleil*, May 20th 2000.
Participate, IFFGD, vol. 8, n° 1, Summer 1999.
Dawn Burstall, R. D., T. Michael Vallis, Ph. D. and Geoffrey K. Turnbull, M. D., *I.B.S. Relief, A doctor, a Dietitian and a Psychologist Provide a Team Approach to Managing Irritable Bowel Syndrome*, Chronimed Publishing, Minneapolis, 176 p.
Qu'est-ce qu'on mange? Le Québec en 820 plats, Les Cercles des Fermières du Québec, vol. 3. 1994.

recommended intake. There are two types of dietary fibres: the soluble fibres, which form a gel when combined with water (groats), and the insoluble ones, which become doughy when added to water (bran). Water-soluble fibres include pectin, which is found in fruits and gums, some vegetables, oats, barley and legumes. Insoluble fibres include lignite (vegetables), cellulose (wheat) and hemicellulose (cereals and vegetables). Several health related characteristics are attributed to soluble fibre, including the reduction of blood cholesterol levels and a slowdown of sugar absorption in the blood. In populations that have a high-fibre diet this characteristic correlates with a low percentage of people suffering from IBS, polyps, hiatus hernia, appendicitis, hemorrhoids and diverticulitis. Both soluble and insoluble fibres slow down intestinal functions that do overtime (reducing diarrhoea), increase the volume of feces as they move into the large intestine (reducing constipation).

The main difficulty of a higher intake of dietary fibre is the gas produced by insoluble fibres. It is recommended to increase them progressively over a long period. Moreover, insoluble fibres absorb up to fifteen times their weight in water, so there is a risk of dehydration and cramps if not enough liquid is taken with the increased fibre.

There are three types of fibre supplements: psyllium, a source of both soluble and insoluble fibres sold in powder form (Hydrocil, Metamucil, Konsyl or Perdiem); methylcellulose, a soluble semi-synthetic fibre that forms a gel but does not ferment (Citrucel, Fibre Naturale); and polycarbophilus, a synthetic fibre that does not ferment (Equalactin, Fibercom). A medical doctor, a pharmacist or dietician can prescribe the supplement best suited to your condition.

A fibre-rich diet takes several weeks to yield results. If your intestine is irritable, any change may cause a flare-up of the symptoms in the short-term.

To reach a level of 20 to 35 g (more on less one once) of fibre daily, you need a high fibre diet requiring you to:

1. consume insoluble fibres (especially from whole-wheat grain);
2. consume an adequate amount of fibre;
3. consume fibre every day;
4. every day, drink eight glasses of water or other non-caffeinated beverages, which can replace a maximum of two glasses of water.

Table XII Fibre content of selected foods		
Nutriments – Portion	Grams	Once
Cereals		
Whole wheat bread (25 g or 1 once slice) – insoluble fibres	1.7	0.06
Bran bread (25 g or 1 once slice) – insoluble fibres	2.1	0.07
Multigrain bread (25 g or 1 once slice) – insoluble fibres	1.8	0.06
Whole wheat muffin (average size) – insoluble fibres	3.8	0.13
Cooked long grain brown rice (120 ml or ½ cup)	1.5	0.05
Cooked whole wheat noodles (120 ml or ½ cup)	2.3	0.08
Cooked oats (250 ml or 1 cup) – soluble fibres	5.7	0.2
Legumes (120 ml or ½ cup)		
Cooked beans – insoluble fibres	9.9	0.35
Cooked dried peas – insoluble fibres	2.9	0.1
Cooked lentils – insoluble fibres	4.3	0.15
Fruits and nuts		
Unbleached dried almonds (10 nuts) – insoluble fibres	1.6	0.06
Banana (average size)	2.0	0.07
Crunchy peanut butter (30 ml or 2 tablespoons)	2.2	0.08

Dates (3) – insoluble fibres	2.0	0.07
Dried figs (3)	9.5	0.34
Apple with skin (average size)	2.6	0.09
Orange (average size)	2.4	0.08
Papaya (average size)	5.3	0.19
Pear with skin left on (average size)	5.0	0.18
Prunes (5)	5.3	0.19
Raisins, (60 ml or ¼ cup); Sultana raisins have a higher fibre content, 9 g per 60 ml or 1/3 once per ¼ cup)	2.5	0.09
Vegetables (120 ml or ½ cup)		
Cooked yellow or green beans – insoluble fibres	1.5	0.05
Cooked lima beans – soluble fibres	4.3	0.15
Cooked Brussels sprouts – soluble fibres	3.4	0.11
Cooked carrot – soluble fibres	2.1	0.07
Raw carrot (moyenne) – soluble fibres	2.0	0.07
Corn (1 ear 30 cm or 1 foot)	6.6	0.23
Cooked green peas – insoluble fibres	3.6	0.13
Cooked potato with skin left on (average size) – soluble fibres	4.5	0.16
Mashed potato – soluble fibres	2.5	0.09
Raw spinach	2.1	0.07
Raw tomato (average size) – soluble fibres	1.5	0.05

Probiotics[73]

Although the term probiotics has existed for the past hundred years, pharmaceutical companies have recently tried to develop and introduce beneficial ingredients in foods, including probiotics. Researcher Aloysius L. D'Souza made an inventory of nine scientific studies dealing with the subject. He concludes that lactobacilli, bifidobacteria and other probiotics have beneficial effects on intestinal flora, especially when combined with antibiotics. They help reduce the period of diarrhoeas and gastroenteritis in children.

Some studies have proven the benefits of L-Plantarium on abdominal pain and bloating, and of VSL3, which seems to work well in the case of bloating. However, according to Dr Bouin, these substances are not necessarily available on the market.

Dr Gregor Reid, of the University of Western Ontario, claims that the survival of a majority of species is due to the balance of bacterial flora in their digestive system. Almost forth of IBS patients suffered a persistent pain following a bacterial infection. It seems that women are three times more susceptible to develop chronic problems after a digestive track bacterial problem. Dr Reid showed that health of laboratory animals exempt from the bacteria is clearly more fragile than the health of their "infested" fellow creatures. Probiotic therapies are animal tested in the dentistry, urinary and surgical fields and used to treat inflammatory intestinal diseases. However, the majority of research is business oriented, and mainly deals with digestive tract microflora. In fact, there are over 400 species of known bacteria in the intestines, and 50 % of fecal matter is made up of these bacteria. In Japan, hundreds of companies have developed probiotics: they

---

[73] D'Souza and others, *Probiotics in prevention of antibiotic associated diarrhea: meta-analysis*. B.M.J., 324 : 1361-4, 2002.
Articles of docteur Philippe Presles, M.D., *E-santé* : http://www.e-sante.fr
Article of Bob Beale, *The Scientist* : http://www.thescientist.com/yr2002/jul/research_020722.html
Jacinthe Côté, Nutritionist, *Le Soleil*, July 4th 2004, p. A 11.

are mainly used to reduce the proliferation of undesirable bacteria in the intestines.

The most widely known probiotics are lactobacilli and bifidobacteria, which are added to yogurts. Kefir also contains various lactic bacteria depending on the recipe (lactobacillus, streptococcus, acetobacter), and yeasts (kluyveromyces, candida, saccharomyces). The authors of IBS for Dummies suggest Lifeway brand for the right kind of kefir. Generally, the intestines resist their introduction, so that there must be a daily intake of these ingredients, which is of great interest to manufacturers. Professor Glenn Gibson of Reading University, in England, predicts that the industry will soon add these bacteria to cheeses, cream and salami, as well as baby formula. The bifidobacteria colonization of the intestinal tract in infants largely explains the undisputed benefits of breastfeeding. These bacteria modify the ambient intestinal acidity and therefore prevent bacterial colonization which causes diarrhoea and gastroenteritis.

It has been suggested that some gastrointestinal infections, including stomach ulcers caused by helicobacter pylori, some diarrhoeas (clostridium difficile) and gastroenteritis, are linked to an imbalance in the gastrointestinal microflora. The pathogenic bacteria imbalance of gastrointestinal microflora appears to promote their development. In this connection, we should mention Escherichia coli; clostridium botulinum, difficile and perfringes; listeria monocytogne; salmonella, campylobacter and vibrio vulnificus. We should also mention the importance of checking the intestinal flora's acidobasic equilibrium. If the diet was modified to restore this balance this would ensure favourable conditions for the growth of beneficial bacteria. Concerning probiotics, there are claims that some of these products protect the flora against pathogenic bacteria. We should point out that the boulardii yeasts (Provultra and Provucal) may be linked to a decrease in the frequency of salmonella and compylobacteria contamination. Apparently, these yeasts are unable to colonize the intestine and their effect is felt as they pass through the gastrointestinal tract to be eliminated through the fecal channel.

Omega-3 [74]

Omega-3, essential fatty nutriments providing food for the brain, are especially rare in the diet of most Occidental countries. A French study on Eskimos, who consume an average of sixteen grams (½ once) of fish oil per day, reveals that in the long term these people produce more neurotransmitters associated with energy and contentment (dopamine) in the emotional brain. Dr Andrew Stoll of Harvard proved the effectiveness of fish oil rich in omega-3 in stabilizing mood and easing depression in manic-depressive patients. Studies conducted by Drs Puri and Nemets tend to show that a wide range of depressive symptoms can be improved by adding omega-3 fatty acids: sadness, lack of energy, anxiety, insomnia, weak libido, suicidal tendencies.

However, Dr Servan-Schreiber points out that we may have to wait several years before a sufficient number of studies of this type are conducted. Since the Omega-3 is taken from nature they are not of great interest to large pharmaceutical companies, especially since their effectiveness may lead to a shrinking demand for antidepressants.

The existing studies suggest that, to obtain an antidepressant effect, one needs to take between two and three grams (0,07 and 0,11 once) a day of a mix of the two fatty acids found in fish: the eicosapentaenoic acid (EPA), which should have the highest content, and the docosahexainoic acid (DHA).

---

[74] David Servan-Schreiber, M. D. et psychiatrist, *Guérir le stress, l'anxiété et la dépression sans médicaments ni psychanalyse*, Robert Laffont, Paris, 2003, chap. IX, p. 145-166.

5 – Various Therapies

• **Physiotherapy**

Physiotherapy, through stretching and muscle strengthening, markedly increases well-being. As opposed to chiropractics, for example, it develops self-sufficiency, which makes it a form of self-treatment. Many exercises such as stretching can be performed at home. However, one should avoid any excess, and persevere.

It is possible to relieve much of the nervous tension lodged in muscles by stretching. Muscular degeneration can be prevented by strengthening exercises. This is the case for people who accumulate too much nervous tension, who become idle due to excess gas, or who regularly suffer from migraines and decrease their activities because of it.

Since I exercise quite a bit, the physical exercises I learned in physiotherapy are of great value to me. I adjust my condition to these activities, and I treat the slightest muscular and articular pain this way. Therefore, especially with cardio exercises, I take advantage of the stirring of the digestive system coming from movements and from deep breathing resulting from my sports activities. I feel that deep breathing associated with physical activities help me to overcome anxiety I experienced when I deep breathe alone.

• Chiropractic

Can chiropractic be helpful when there is locking of the spinal joints, or to treat migraines caused by a faulty alignment of cervical vertebrae? In my case, it was in the first months of treatment that chiropractic was the most effective. Later on the treatments would leave me with recurring pain in the hips. I felt a great release of energy in the abdomen but I also got the impression that it triggered an attack of gas. When my body was not as strong, in my early thirties, a combination of chiropractic-physiotherapy gave excellent results. I no longer turn to chiropractic and continue to do my physiotherapy exercises. Like Dr Barrett, of Quackwatch, I do not appreciate the dependency this discipline entails.

• Acupuncture

Dr David Servan-Schreiber devotes a chapter of his book to acupuncture. According to the Institute of Tibetan Medicine, emotional and physical symptoms are two aspects of an underlying imbalance of energy flow called Qi (pronounce chi). There are three ways of influencing the Qi: meditation, which regenerates the Qi, diet and medicinal herbs and, the most direct one, acupuncture. The World Health Organization recognizes acupuncture as an accepted, effective medical practice. Over time, its effectiveness has been recognized for treating a growing number of ailments including migraine, depression, anxiety, insomnia and intestinal problems. Dr Hui, with his team of the Masachusetts General Hospital, has shown that acupuncture could be aimed directly at the emotional brain. One Harvard study demonstrated that the needles can block the areas in the emotional brain responsible for feelings of pain and anxiety. Another benefit of acupuncture is its influence on the equilibrium between the two branches of the autonomous nervous system (the sympathetic and parasympathetic nervous systems).

However, another study conducted by Dr Klaus Linde, published in the Journal of the American Medical Association, indicates that acupuncture is effective regardless of the area where the needles are inserted, which indicates a strong placebo effect, or non specific effect, produced by the needles. This hypothesis has also been confirmed by another study (Schneider, Gut 2006; 55: 649-654) mentioned on Egora (www.egora.fr), conducted with two groups of patients suffering from IBS, one group having been treated by acupuncture and the other, by "placebo" acupuncture. In both groups there was a significant improvement of the overall quality of life when the treatment was completed. However, three months later this effect had vanished. The prevailing effect was a better adaptation to everyday life.

• Antigymnastic

After training in antigymnastic, my wife introduced me to the discipline. This is a type of soft gymnastics (not always, because you can go overboard and cause an inflammation), which is very effective in relieving muscle tension. The stretchings and use of balls make the self-treatment of the back, neck and shoulders easier. Small hard balls are used for a deep, more specific treatment. Antigymnastic helps us assess the level of muscle tension.

The principle of antigymnastic is fairly simple and consistent with the release of nervous tension. When sustained pressure is applied on a muscle it eventually relaxes. The way it works is: balls are used to apply pressure along the muscles without exerting any direct pressure on the vertebrae or joints. The level and duration of the pressure on the muscle being treated can be adjusted. A good session lasts approximately thirty minutes. In my case, I start with two balls and apply pressure on the buttock muscles on both sides of the coccyx because they are the largest muscles of the body and, when they are relaxed, it helps ensure muscular balance on the entire back. Every thirty seconds or so I move the balls a few centimetres or an inch at a time along the back muscles. I finish with the trapezius muscles, and the muscles of the neck and nape of the neck. The balls used for antigymnastic are specific to this discipline, but in my case I use tennis balls because they adhere well to clothing (stability) and, with practice after a while, their firmness no longer causes acute pain.

This is one of my favourite techniques, which I practice regularly, even when I am at the office. It is also part of a self-treatment approach.

• Psychotherapy

My psychoanalysis allowed me to discover the significance of language, and of the connection between the body and psychological tensions. Some people postulate that the slowness and excessive sensitivity of the intestinal tract is caused by an inclination to hold back, to give nothing. We can avoid all the attitudes, thoughts, habits that cause such holding back. However, we can try to reduce the psychological tensions that are self-imposed, with our "we must", "they did this to me", "I should", "because of my past", etc. We can also improve our quality of life by making decisions and resolutions that are suitable for us. We can also learn to become more assertive in our environment and towards ourselves, accept our imperfections, and realize that other people can provide feedback and help us reduce our social tension level, and therefore our inner tension.

One studied approach is hypnotherapy. A 2003 a study published in the journal *Gut* found 71 percent of patients responded well initially to hypnotherapy[75]. Of that number, 81 percent maintained their improvement over 5 years, and the other relapsed only slightly. The subjects had fewer doctors' visits, less medication, and much less anxiety and depression.

I have to insist on the usefulness of psychotherapy because the fact that I regularly release gas and excess nervous tension has greatly changed the way I perceive my well-being, my abilities and my holding back. That gave me enough interior space to treat my

---

[75] IBS for Dummies, p. 117.

psychological tensions. This is on my view, one of the good side effects of my exercises.

Expressing our personality by working on the consequences (pay now, get the benefits later) is similar to managing our stools adequately. We need to "let go" right now and hope that we will be rewarded with an improvement in our physiological and psychological availability, which should result in a more satisfactory quality of life. We must act as if we functioned properly, but without feeling that the cost will be too high. Working on the "economics" of somatisation also allows me to find benefits in "investing" in myself.

Pharmaceutical and relational dependency is similar to the relationship we sometimes have with our gastrointestinal system. By holding ourselves in to avoid suffering, the pains accumulate as the gas developing in a sluggish system. This leads to more retention to control the pain — or so we think. We can then fall victims of our need to protect ourselves against the pain.

Gastrointestinal discomfort arising from relational problems in early childhood can explain many of our inner conflicts. Rebellion, power struggles and jalousie are often fallout of gastric problems. I don't feel well and I won't take it lying down! The inner and relational conflicts become a kind of favourite behavioural scheme that we cannot readily escape from. Studying our schemes or automatic reflexes as they relate to our social or private relationships is an important step. For example, constantly clashing with authority often has serious consequences in terms of physiological discomfort, stress in addition to limiting our social life. "Chronic fear makes you breathe shallowly and suck in your intestines and tighten them up. After a while, you don't even know you're doing it.[76]"

We can work on consequences, on improving our "relationships", on starting each day by putting our best foot forward: this should help us build muscle tone, improve circulation and abdominal activity.

---

[76] Ibid, p. 119.

Those who have already started or would like to start psychotherapy should know that to loosen up you need to work on the body. I was able to experiment that the resistance phases tended to fade following intense work on the body. However, I don't think that the release of gas and excess nervous tension can be considered a cure-all. If we do not take advantage of this method to make other changes in our lives, in our activities, in our attitudes and in our projects, the release of gas and excess nervous tension alone can become tiresome and eventually be neglected.

Most psychotherapy can help to put words, so self awareness and care, on particular physical pain or even illness we could experiment. In my view, this also could become a form self treatment approach.

• Neurolinguistic programming

Considering how useful it can be to learn different modes of expression, neurolinguistics is widely used in this connection. Neurolinguistics is based on the concept of cognitive distortion. Any reflection or expression of reality is basically a subjective exercise. Out of habit, preference or education, we tend to favour thought patterns that move away quite a bit from the reality they try to explain. The expression of our discomfort should not be worse that what caused it. In the realm of neurolinguistics, our interpretation of reality determines what we feel. For example, according to neurolinguistics, depression is not what makes us interpret life in a "depressing" way, but it is rather the way in which we interpret life that is eventually depressing. Therefore, it seems that health is achieved by the smooth management of our interpretative or expressive activities.

Although I have not experienced neurolinguistic programming myself, I am convinced that it can bring relief or at least a more open outlook. It then becomes possible to choose the type of emotion we wish to experience and adjust our interpretative habits to achieve this goal. We can learn to express ourselves, turn things in our mind so that we may be less uptight, or somatise less. Neurolinguistics therefore belongs to the self-treatment approach.

• Emotional Freedom Techniques[77] (EFT)

Christine Wheeler, one of the authors of IBS for Dummies (www. christinewheeler.com) is an EFT practitioner. Gary Craig the founder of ETF (www.emofree.com) says that the cause of any physical illness is one of two things: a disruption in the body's energy system, or unresolved emotional trauma. You must choose the problem you want to work on. For example, *I have IBS*. Then you scale the discomfort it causes from 1 to 10 (10 being very intense). You must insert your problem into this affirmative statement: "Even though I have IBS (problem), I deeply and completely accept myself." Then you combine loud repetition of the reminder of the sentence (here: "I have IBS") with tapping of the "Karate Chop" point on the fleshy part on the side of either hand. The tapping and repeating have to be made on 8 other acupuncture points six or seven times each. After that process, you check back in the discomfort rating of the problem. Like any technique the success comes from persistence. So you must practice up to the point until you feel like you have dissolved the problem.

For example, in case of pain, the problem could be: "Pain is frightening." the setup phrase: "Even though this pain is scary, I deeply and completely accept myself." and the reminder phrase: "Pain is scary." A non endorsed list of EFT practitioner is available on Gary Graig's Web site.

• The place occupied by the conscious and the subconscious

The concept of subconscious, propagated by Freud, describes a part of the personality which is relatively inaccessible to the conscious, which possesses a deep-seated memory, is governed by the pleasure

---

[77] Ibid, pp. 214-225.

principle and finds expression through somatisation, misactions and various perversions of the personality. The superego, also lodged in the subconscious, represents what some would call a deeply buried "bad father" who constantly makes us feel guilty without caring for our happiness or health.

It is easier in life to let our subconscious take over. Our subconscious often expresses its displeasure, or rather tries to compensate for its dissatisfaction, through the body. In its own way it maintains that our whole being needs pleasure to survive. If the ego becomes helpless because of the demands of the superego and cannot express itself satisfactorily in real life, the subconscious comes along and finds its own pleasures, and people can find themselves weighed down by sensations, behaviours, a character they will fall victims to. Psychoanalysis allows us to move forward on the difficult road to self-knowledge. We have to find out what we are burdening our bodies with and what we can assume consciously. The ego is then better prepared to choose its rewards, the pleasures that can bridge the gap between the conscious and the subconscious, and make peace between them. For the subconscious, taking over is not something pleasant, consciously or not, so it must find some compensation.

It is probably impossible to be entirely conscious or to achieve perfect peace between the conscious and the subconscious. We should realize how convenient it is to have subconscious as well as functioning habits. We can analyze them and negotiate what we are unable to change. Although a large part of our personality or functioning remains at the subconscious level, studying the consequences of our automatic reflexes, vicious circles or bad habits allows us to assess the cost of relying too much on the subconscious. We can then try to express ourselves in a more satisfying manner.

Here I would quote from the words of Henry G. Tietze on the importance of taking responsibility for ourselves:

"The day we feel that we are running in circles and that nothing new is happening in our lives, it is important to do some soul-searching. It is essential, then, to take stock of our lives and compare assets and liabilities, if we hope to ever free ourselves from old habits that threaten our existence, and make room for new experiences.

Because, how can we be happy when we are grappling with feelings that have been repressed deep inside? No, and this is why the road to consciousness is the only one that can lead us to freedom, even though it may be heavy going. We may be sure that any introspection brings up to the surface negative emotions that have always been deeply repressed.

However, the most unpleasant part of our task is not to "dig up these dead bodies" deeply buried in our subconscious, but rather to carry out a "post-mortem" revealing their true nature so that we may stop them from intimidating us any longer.

Now, we've learned not to look directly at things. Yet, to free ourselves from our past we must have that courage. To become a visionary, we have to keep our eyes wide open. It is the only way we can acquire true knowledge, knowledge that leads to righteous action and, through it, to freedom."

The accumulation of nervous tension and gas can be part of the economics of the personality. It can therefore also rob us of our "freedom". As you know, psychoanalysis can go on for life. But I don't think it has to be a life sentence. I went to my analysis for six years and, even though I do not assume it is completed, I remind many inside dead bodies that came alive and have been assumed and, more importantly, how I can continue to do so. In this regard, this could be part of a self treatment approach.

- **Colonic irrigation** [78]

The main purpose of colonic irrigation is to void the cæcum, the part of the large intestine that comes after the small intestine, or "bottom" of the colon. One of the treatments consists in getting in and out of the colon – by means of a mechanical device with two tubes – fifteen to twenty litres or pints of pure water with a neutral Ph, heated to 35 degrees Celcius. The patient is not required to push out or hold in the water. The cæcum is reached through a siphon effect. In another technique, hot water alternates with cold water to stimulate the muscle tone of the intestinal wall and strengthen it. The content of the caecum is then ejected through peristaltic movements. There will then be an attempt to restore the intestinal flora by the use of acidophilus bacterial supplements, the normal balance of the so-called "friendly" bacteria (85 %) and "enemy" bacteria (15 %). It is a fairly common occurrence to need ten to twenty irrigations. The inoculation of sunflower or linseed oil, as well as a daily intake of fibre, also guarantees that the benefits of the treatment will be fully felt. To these treatments are added the benefits of naturopathy, in which roughage, germinations, greens, fruits and the proper food combinations can play a significant role.

According to Dr Michel Boivin, gastroenterologist at the Hôpital Saint-Luc, the hygienists' theory is not in the least scientific (refer to the site Passeportsante.net). According to him, there is nothing harmful in the colon; it is a tank that receives material that has not been absorbed during normal digestion. "The bacteria grab hold of this material, metabolize it and feed on it to give us back the energy we lost during digestion. It is the only place in the digestive tract where fermentation occurs, the colon is a kind of ecosystem where

---

[78]   http://www.passeportsante.net/fr/therapies/guide/articleinteret.aspx? doc=hygiene_colon_montpetit_f_1992_th from an article by Francine Montpetit published in *Guide Ressources*, vol. 7, n° 6, 1992, p. 28-35. http://www.allerg.qc.ca/charlgastro.htm : « *Le charlatanisme gastro-intestinal : coloniques, laxatifs, et plus* ».

bacteria proliferate allowing us to digest and protect ourselves from outside attacks. Washing is like washing clean clothes!"

He adds that, "if the colon doesn't work well, we get the impression that it is paralyzed. This is not the case. We also get the feeling that it changes shape and collapses. This is not true either! In my view, the colon cannot become encrusted, as hygienists maintain. The particles loosened during a treatment are usually stool residues lodged in small pockets that do not cause any damage, even though they may have been there for years. Instead, the bloating should be attributed to a poor coordination of intestinal movements. In short, not everything can be treated through the colon. There is also a risk, although minor, of infection or trauma from the insertion of the tube in the rectum, a risk of lesions, of anal fistulas, hemorrhoids, stenoses and diverticules. Moreover, some people do not tolerate large quantities of liquid in the colon (heart or kidney patients). Finally, the views held by colonic hygienists are not acceptable when they make outlandish promises. Unfortunately, it is easier to have irrigation than to take responsibility for our lives and get the machine going."

Naturally, these apprehensions do not hold water for the advocates of this practice, who earn their living performing colonic irrigation. According to psychologist Louise Noiseux, constipation, which is the main reason invoked by patients for turning to colonic irrigation, symbolizes a refusal of authority, a refusal to function. In life there are all kinds of authorities, there is the school, our boss, our spouse, and we can even go as far as to impose this retention on ourselves. We say "no" for all sorts of reasons and finally, we no longer feel anything. We end up so emotionally and physically cramped that we no longer control our intestines and viscera.

Dr Barrett, founder of Quackwatch, mentions the position of the California Health Department's Infectious Disease Branch, which warns that "the practice of colon irrigation by chiropractors, physical therapists or physicians must stop. Colonic irrigation does nothing good, only harm."

I have never had colonic irrigation and I do not intend to try it. As you know, in my case, once my stomach has been evacuated my large intestine systematically recovers its tonus. This restores the flatulence movements, and the evacuation is done "cleanly."

• Relaxation (a few existing techniques)

To express ourselves, many specialists recommend lowering stress level, developing self-knowledge and learning to be consciously self-assertive by using words instead of the body. When practiced on a regular basis, relaxation techniques, including transcendental meditation, yoga and prayer, help calm the digestive system and promote gas release. These techniques also reduce nervous tension build-up and help us become more self-focused. They can also heighten our perception and help us understand the kind of stress we have experienced in the last few hours or days.

If the physical attacks appear during our relaxation technique, we should let them pass (express it) as much as possible. However, these attacks can be turned into something positive, in the sense that they can help reduce the tension built up in our body. It also reveals the importance of making changes in our lives, thoughts and expectations, and also of finding means to release the tension we tend to repress.

These relaxation activities can also be viewed as a break, as a time unlike any other we usually experience. Here are a few excerpts from a book by Dr Yves Lamontagne (Techniques de relaxation, France Amérique, 1982):

"... the Quinodoz procedure seems very sensible to us: 'When a person who comes to me for a consultation situates his or her demand below the language level, I usually suggest relaxation; when it is at the language level, I prefer to abandon the idea of relaxation and use instead the elaboration that speech allows.

If the therapist knows various relaxation techniques, the procedure we have developed can be useful. When it is indicated to learn a relaxation technique, we teach an active technique such as progressive relaxation in cases where the patient's anxiety level is so high that the clinician feels that there is a psychological risk of emotional collapse. An active relaxation method lets the patient stay in touch with reality and it causes far less anxiety, side-effects and complications than other relaxation techniques. With all other patients for whom relaxation is advisable we use a passive method, most of the time self-generated training, either by itself or combined with biofeedback training. The combination of these two treatments is often beneficial, at least in the beginning, as we were able to show in one of our research projects. In fact, biofeedback training allows the patient to learn to relax easily and rapidly, and the self-generated training exercises done at home add to the improvement experienced in the biofeedback laboratory. Finally, we still use hypnosis on rare occasions, sometimes when all other techniques have failed, and in the case of highly dependent subjects who refuse to do relaxation techniques on their own. Hypnosis may give rapid results in some cases.

Before you begin doing a relaxation technique you should choose the one that appeals to you the most, as well as a good trainer.

There are significant differences among individuals as far as the duration of relaxation training, which varies according to the age and habits of the subjects, the regularity of training sessions, the ability to follow instructions faithfully and, naturally, and the type of problem that needs to be rectified. Generally, in the case of anxiety, a three to six-month period of strict training will yield benefits for the subject, whatever the relaxation technique learned.

Jacobson relates that any effort to relax inevitably causes the failure of the process. Adopting a passive attitude when one is learning a relaxation technique is probably the key thing. The following instructions can be useful in achieving this goal: relaxation should not be forced, let it come to you. Do not concern yourself with achieving a good or bad performance. If your attention is distracted, it doesn't necessarily mean that you are not doing it right, but if it happens, simply repeat the sentences used in your relaxation technique, if any, and stop worrying.

Finally, we cannot put too much emphasis on the importance of a daily routine to learn relaxation habits and really experience the effects of relaxation. If the subject neglects the exercises they risk losing what they have already gained; besides, the big problem is that people stop practicing their relaxation technique as soon as they feel they've experienced positive effects. We must remember that only by accomplishing these exercises regularly, rigorously and steadfastly can we ensure our progress and the durable effects of the learning process. On average, the exercises should be done one to three times a day; their duration depends on the technique used."

Prayer also appears to be an excellent relaxation method, for letting go and asking for help. In a television program describing the life of a hundred-year-old nun, we learned that she prayed for half an hour both morning and night. I often turn to prayer when my relaxation techniques lead to an anxiety attack or intense pain. It enables me to accept, endure and find relief more rapidly. Praying also means asking God to help and guide us. We then contribute more actively to our own well-being, regain our self-confidence and let go; it is as if we admitted to ourselves that we cannot solve everything on our own.

A 2001 study on IBS at State University of New York[79] showed that after six-week period, participants using a relaxation response reported significant improvements in symptoms of diarrhoea, belching, bloating, and flatulence.

• Other sources of help[80]

A lot of information is available on IBS on the Web. This section is to provide information – not endorsements – so, once again, I encourage you to be discerning. The Web information and groups are not substitute for a consultation with an appropriate medical professional.

Many organizations have Web site, support groups and newsletter : Canadian Society of Intestinal Research (www.badgut.com);

---

[79] IBS for Dummies, p. 226.
[80] Idem, pp. 329-338.

International Foundation for Functional Gastrointestinal Disorders (www.iffgd.org); Irritable Bowel Syndrome Association (in the U.S. : www.ibsassociation.org , in Canada : www.ibsassociation.ca); and in French, the *Association québécoise pour les maladies gastro-intestinales fonctionnelles* (www.mauxdeventre.org). There is also the IBS Self Help and Support Group like www.ibsgroup.org, which claims to be the largest online patient advocate and support community for people with IBS.

For exercise resources, you can find the site of Theresa Tapp (www.t-tapp.com), the Yoga Journal (www.yogajournal.com) and Yoga Basics (www.yogabasics.com) and the technique Nadeau site (http://www.techniquenadeau.com), which I recommend the practice.

For the gluten intolerance or celiac disease, you may found the Canadian Celiac Association (www.celiac.ca), the Celiac Disease and Gluten-free Diet Support Center (www.celiac.com) and the Celiac Disease Foundation (www.celiac.org). For inflammatory bowel disease (IBD), there is Crohn's & Colitis Foundation of America (www.ccfa.org); and for lactose intolerance (www.lactose.co.uk).

For herbal medicine you may find information in the site of American Botanical Council (www.herbalgram.org) and the Herb Research Foundation (www.herbs.org).

6 – CONCLUSION

This book describes the natural exercises I do to release gas and nervous tension. These exercises help improve my general well-being noticeably while also helping to move gas through the digestive system. The exercises also reduce the frequency and intensity of many IBS related symptoms and help treat them rapidly.

However, there are difficulties associated with the exercises, such as increased discomfort in the early stages of gas release, isolation (accepting the fact that we cannot always be comfortable with or benefit from the presence of others, or be useful to them), regularly having to go back and redo the exercises. To yield positive results, my approach requires developing and maintaining a relatively high level of consciousness and curiosity about ourselves. We also need to accept the fact that our symptoms may result from the way we function.

We may also have to come to terms with the fact that we may not be like everyone; we have to take this in and tell ourselves that life is perhaps more painful for us but that we can improve our condition. And that we should not give in to depression or self-indulgence.

I also find it difficult to communicate these techniques without some kind of therapeutic support. I don't know of any trainers, although I dream of being able to train some myself one day.

However, experienced therapists can probably test these methods and adapt them to the patient's needs and capabilities. The book IBS for Dummies suggests the creation of IBS clinics which could offer several non-invasive tests to determine whether what we experience is food intolerance or allergy: hydrogen breath tests to check for lactose intolerance; blood antibody tests to check for gluten intolerance; and blood tests to determine food allergies. These clinics could be a good place to teach my techniques.

Over and above a description of my approach, one of my goals for this book was to provide useful information on existing IBS treatments. The aim is to help prepare readers for their own approach, whether they try it solo or with the help of health care professionals. Writing the review of literature required a great deal of work. I feel that information is a key component of the self-treatment approach.

I wish to thank you, dear reader, because you are the main justification for all the efforts I put into this book, and for the efforts I will probably devote to it in the future, depending on its success.

Finally, I hope that many people will have a chance of experiencing the "freedom" provided by the release of gas and excess nervous tension. It is only to that extent that I will have realized one of my dreams, help people, if only to chase away their "inner winds."

Larry Tremblay,
June 12 2011.

ANNEXE I

My child has a bellyache

Children are vulnerable to abdominal pain that often becomes uncomfortable (nausea, insomnia, cramps, excitement). Abdominal pain, like sleep deprivation, can result from numerous causes, including some that require a visit to the doctor (when there is a fever, persistent pain, etc.) For example, when very young a child needs to develop the oral tolerance process[81], which means that his or her digestive system must adapt to the absorption of a foreign body (antigen) or an allergenic substance without setting the entire immune system into action. An antigen is any substance that excites immune system enough to produce antibodies to fight against it. For instance, between 2 and 6% of all Occidental newborn babies are allergic to the protein (casein, beta-lactoglobulin, etc.) generally found in cow's milk. Over half of these children will suffer from gastrointestinal disorders or cutaneous reactions, and a third will have respiratory problems. Nowadays, it is admitted that it is the digestive system which is responsible for nearly 80 % of the immune defence functions, resulting mainly from the presence of lymphatic tissue and friendly bacteria colonies.

Recurrent abdominal pain is the most common pain complaint of childhood. A study showed that one-third to one-half of children

---

[81]   Jacinthe Côté, in *Le Soleil*, January 23th, 2005, page A-10

with recurrent abdominal pain continues to report it and related symptoms when they are adults[82]. Children haven't developed adult coping skills and they tend to put up with the pain (passive coping) or they can feel victimized by the pain (castratrophyzing). There are many things you can do to install confidence in you child. You can let him know that his feelings are important, and that you will always support him. Avoiding trigger foods like ice cream, cereals with sugar added, candies, chips, must be strictly managed.

However, most of the time, children's abdominal pain is not considered to be a serious disorder. In older children it often results from a poor diet (too much sugar, starch, chips or sodas), stress (school related, small hurts, and important changes), heat (dehydration) or simply a response to a virus or an antibiotic.

I rely on the assumption that children, even older ones, may need help to let out a burp, like infants do. All mothers know that an infant, who hasn't been burped or not burped sufficiently, is bound to get colicky and have a restless sleep.

To help children release troublesome gas before putting them to bed:

1. Make sure the child is well hydrated;
2. Tickle the child to make him or her laugh (not too much to avoid hurting or overexciting the child);
3. Sit him on your knees or next to you (when the child is older) and rock him gently… until he naturally lets out a small belch;
4. Repeat exercise number 3, lifting the child's knees to his stomach (excellent for releasing intestinal gas);
5. Lay the child on his stomach over your knee and gently pat him (or take him in your arms and pat him on the back).

---

[82]   IBS for Dummies, p. 264-266.

6. Smaller children can be laid face down over your shoulder and held head first while you pace up and down in the house (dads really enjoy this!);
7. When the child lets out a belch and, if necessary, a little fart put him to bed on his stomach.
8. Two-year-olds and over should always be given encouragement when they belch or fart: later on adjustments can be made for when you are with other people.

For best results you can alternate between one minute of exercises in 3 or 4 and one minute of exercises in 5. Repeat three or four times, it should be enough. Chances are that the child will sleep better and recuperate well. In the long run, the child may even maintain a flexible digestive system with no excess tension. If the child often has abdominal pain a doctor should be consulted, his or her dietary balance should be checked, and foods that promote gas production or which the child cannot tolerate should be reduced.

A simple relaxation technique

Before putting a child to bed it is useful to get them to relax. We can develop the good habit of reading or singing a lullaby to the child. For relaxation, here is a technique that worked well with my own child when he was between the ages of five and eight.

First, use a short ritual sentence that will be repeated between your appeals for relaxation. Naturally, the terms used can vary from one child, or one parent, to the next. The one that works best for me is this:

Put the child to bed and tell him softly: "One, two, three, four... Get your belly real soft!"

Lay your hand on the child's abdomen to check its degree of relaxation. At first, check this regularly. Once the habit is well installed, check occasionally to make sure it is maintained.

Then, repeat the ritual sentence, asking the child to relax his or her legs, back, shoulders, arms, neck, head, etc. This also allows the child to become aware of the various body parts and to learn how to relax them.

It is useful to check the child's breathing for any modifications. Deeper breathing is a sign that he or she is about to go to sleep. The exercise can then be suspended and you can wish the child good night.

ANNEXE II

A guide for "Happy Holidays"

Some claim that the digestive system is a second brain because it contains the largest number of nervous cells next to the cerebral cortex. The challenge of the holiday period is to prevent the problems of the second brain to become the priority of the first one. Here are a few tips developed over the years by someone who has a fairly delicate system.

Alcoholic beverages: drink lots of fluids before and after you drink alcohol since alcohol usually causes dehydration. You will drink less, eliminate better, and above all, avoid the bilious attack of the morning after.

Hearty meals: why not eliminate hearty meals by preparing delicious appetizers, washed down with alcohol, and followed by a dessert. This may help avoid a salmonellosis caused by leftovers from the main course, including inadequately stored poultry. If you wish to maintain the hearty main course tradition, avoid desserts or reduce the number of meals to two a day instead of three.

Avoid eating before bedtime: going to sleep with a full stomach often exposes one to abdominal pain including gastroesophageal reflux, bloating and weight gain.

Make sure to exercise: taking a walk after drinking your coffee and liqueur is a real tonic. Being sedentary and overeating can be detrimental to your health.

Do not "hold yourself in": things such as travel or entertaining, or not being able to find a rest room when you need it may interfere with your ability to relieve yourself when you feel the need. The body does not always adjust well to this kind of retention.

Renew with spiritual tradition: religious practice during the holidays allows us, at the very least, to spend a few hours without drinking or eating. We often tend to behave decently before Mass or the New Year's Day blessing, indeed a health benefit.

Give yourself some leeway since socializing can cause havoc with the abdomen. I feel that the members of one's family, even if we dearly love them, are people who have been imposed upon us over a long period. If you plan to entertain or visit people for a number of days, you can always say that you have something planned mid-way into the party and you don't know if this will take place or not. You are not obligated to mention your need to recuperate. Another way to avoid abuse is to reduce the number of visits.

Gas release: what better way to release gas than to perform these exercises before travelling or visiting the family? A discreet stroll in the garden or retiring to a quiet place for a few minutes to perform them will let you cheerfully recuperate, leaving some "space" for what will follow.

Update the health care services information: inquire about the opening hours of the various clinics in the area you visit, this is reassuring and will help you avoid the long hours spent in a jam-packed emergency. If you take medication, stock up on them before leaving for a holiday to avoid having to run to the drugstore at any hour.

May your second brain keep your first one happy!

APPENDIX III

TO DATE, YOUR TECHNIQUE IS THE MOST EFFECTIVE IN BRINGING ME SOME RELIEF.
MR SAMSON, BAIE-COMEAU, QUÉBEC.

MANY THANKS FOR YOUR BOOK. I CONGRATULATE YOU FOR WRITING IT.
MR ACCATINO, GRENOBLE, FRANCE.

I STARTED READING IT AND I AM FASCINATED...
MRS NOËL, OTTAWA, ONTARIO.

THANKS FOR YOUR BOOK AND YOUR COMPASSION FOR PEOPLE WITH HEALTH PROBLEMS.
MRS DESMEULES, ANCIENNE-LORETTE, QUÉBEC.

I HAVE STARTED FREEING MYSELF AND I ALREADY SEE AN IMPROVEMENT. I AM VERY GRATEFUL TO YOU FOR THIS.
MRS DESNOYERS, BEAUPORT, QUÉBEC.

THANK YOU FOR YOUR HELP. YOUR BOOK IS INTERESTING, EVEN MORE SO SINCE LITTLE HAS BEEN WRITTEN ON IBS.
MRS GIROUX, QUÉBEC, QUÉBEC.

YOUR BOOK WAS VERY HELPFUL TO ME. AFTER I UNDERWENT A GASTROSCOPY AND AN ENDOSCOPY, I HAD CRAMPS AND LOTS OF GAS. I THOUGHT I WOULD HAVE TO FORCE MYSELF TO BELCH, BUT THE BELCHES CAME AUTOMATICALLY. AFTER TWO OR THREE DAYS I HAD NO MORE GAS. THANK YOU FOR DARING TO SHARE WITH OTHERS SOMETHING WHICH MAY SEEM ECCENTRIC ON THE SURFACE.
MRS BOULANGER, LONGUEUIL, QUÉBEC.

I LEARNED QUITE A BIT ABOUT THE PROBLEMS... FOR WHICH THE HEALTH CARE PROFESSIONALS I CONSULTED HAVE BEEN HELPLESS TO DATE. YOUR BOOK IS A SOURCE OF INFORMATION OF GREAT VALUE.
MR BÉLANGER, OTTAWA, ONTARIO.

IT IS TO YOUR CREDIT THAT YOU HAVE ACCUMULATED LOTS OF INFORMATION. I CONGRATULATE YOU FOR THIS AND THANK YOU FOR SHARING IT WITH US.
MRS LEBLANC, MONTRÉAL, QUÉBEC.

SINCE I WAS BROUGHT UP PROPERLY I NEVER DARED DO WHAT IS DESCRIBED IN YOUR BOOK! SO, I MUST CONVINCE MYSELF DO THE EXERCISES... NOT THAT EASY...
MRS PRÉVOST, SAINT-JÉRÔME, QUÉBEC.

I HOPE TO MAKE THE MOST OF YOUR EXPERIENCE AND YOUR RESEARCH, BUT IN AND OF ITSELF, YOUR TESTIMONIAL IS ENCOURAGING.
MR COULOMBE, SAINT-JEAN-PORT-JOLI, QUÉBEC.

... I LEARNED IN YOUR BOOK SEVERAL EXERCISES THAT I FOUND HELPFUL...
MRS D'ANJOU, SEPT-ÎLES, QUÉBEC.

I THOUGHT THAT I WOULD BE DIFFERENT DURING MY ENTIRE LIFE WHEN MY DOCTOR TOLD ME THAT THERE WAS NO CURE FOR COLOPATHY. THANKS TO YOUR BOOK I WILL CERTAINLY KNOW MYSELF BETTER AND THEREFORE ALLEVIATE THE ATTACKS.
MR LE BRAS, LANDIVISIAU, FRANCE.

THANK YOU, THIS BOOK ALLOWED ME TO BEAR MY LAST ATTACK WITHOUT LOSING HOPE. I HAVE MORE POWER, I CAN RELIEVE MY PAIN.
MRS MATTE, OUTREMONT, QUÉBEC.

DO YOU REMEMBER THE MILD WEATHER WE ENJOYED IN SEPTEMBER 2000 AND THE VERY TASTY APPLES THAT CAME TO US AT THE TIME! THANKS TO YOUR EXERCISES I WAS ONCE AGAIN ABLE TO BITE INTO THIS FRUIT THAT HAD BEEN "FORBIDDEN" TO ME. IMAGINE HOW PLEASED AND HAPPY I WAS... MY HEARTFELT THANKS.
MRS RODRIGUE, POINTE-LEBEL, QUÉBEC.

THIS BOOK HAS HELPED ME TO "BECOME INTROSPECTIVE" AND FIND OUT THE REASONS FOR MY ILL-BEING. FROM NOW ON I REALLY LEARNED TO MAKE FRIEND WITH MY BODY AND NO LONGER TORTURE IT, BUT QUITE THE REVERSE, SUPPORT IT IN HEALTH AND SERENITY.

AT FIRST I READ IT VERY QUICKLY AND LET A FEW DAYS PASS... IT HAD TOUCHED SOME NERVES AND MY "TABOOS"... FOR YEARS DOCTORS KEPT TELLING ME THAT I WAS "FULL OF AIR," BUT I HAD NEVER MADE THE CONNECTION, AND THEY DID NOT GIVE ME ANY ADVICE! LITTLE BY LITTLE, I DID THE EXERCISES. PREVIOUSLY, MY ABDOMEN WAS "IN MY HEAD" SO ALLOWING MYSELF TO SIMPLY "BE" WAS DIFFICULT!

THEN I PICKED UP THE BOOK AGAIN AND UNDERLINED IN YELLOW ALL THE SENTENCES THAT HAD MEANING FOR ME, AND I WAS BETTER ABLE TO ASSIMILATE THE TEXTS AND THE APPENDICES.

I RECOGNIZED MYSELF IN THE BOOK BECAUSE I WAS BROUGHT UP VERY RIGIDLY, MY FATHER TERRORIZED ME AND I HAD NO SUPPORT WHATSOEVER FROM MY MOTHER. IF I WAS TO SUMMARIZE MY CHILDHOOD IN ONE WORD, IT WOULD BE: FEAR! MY PARENTS WERE PROUD OF HOW THEY WERE RAISING THEIR CHILDREN! AND THEY WERE EVEN CONGRATULATED FOR IT... WE DID NOT "MOVE" AND WERE STRICTLY OBEDIENT. AT THE TIME, UNFORTUNATELY, MY FATHER CONFUSED A HOME WITH MILITARY BARRACKS!

I WAS IN THERAPY FOR OVER TEN YEARS, MY FATHER IS NOW AN ELDERLY 82-YEAR-OLD MAN AND I FORGAVE HIM, BUT SO MUCH DAMAGE WAS DONE!

I FOUND AN ECHO OF MY LIFE IN MUCH OF WHAT YOU SAID IN YOUR BOOK, FOR ME IT HAS BEEN LIKE A DIFFICULT STRUGGLE RATHER THAN FLOWING RIVER!
MRS MARION, BESANÇON, FRANCE.

BIBLIOGRAPHY

Agora online medical magazine : http://www.agora.fr

Association des maladies gastro-intestinales fonctionnelles (AMGIF) :
Pamphlets : *RGO - Le reflux gastro-œsophagien; La dyspepsie non
ulcéreuse; SII – Syndrome de l'intestin irritable – renseignements
destinés aux patients.* : www.mauxdeventre.org

Bailey, Robert. Naoki Chiba, Keith G. Tolman, Richard N. Fedorak,
Stephen Wolman, Stepen Sontag, Pamela Rose. Supplement.
In *Le Clinicien – La revue de formation médicale continue,* STA
communications Inc., November 1995.

Baribeau, Hélène. November 2000. In *Guide ressources,* pp. 24 - 27.

Beale, Bob. 2002. *The Scientist* : http://www.thescientist.com/
yr2002/jul/research_020722.html

Bernard, Edmont-Jean. December 1996. *Helicobacter pylori et ulcères
gastro-duodénaux. Le Clinicien – La revue de formation médicale
continue,* STA communications Inc., Vo 11, no 12, pp. 63 - 78.

Bouin, Mickael. Winter 2005. *La constipation fonctionnelle : un
symptôme unique pour des mécanismes multiples.* In *Du cœur au ventre,*
AMGIF. pp. 2 -3.

Bradette, Marc. M. D., Octobre 2003. *Le syndrome du côlon irritable : ce que vous devez savoir. Le Clinicien,* V. 18, n° 10. : http://www. stacommunications.com/journals/leclinicien/archive2003.html

Bradette, Marc. Gastroentirologist, February 2002. In *Le Médecin du Québec,* FMOQ. V. 37. No 2. http://www.fmoq.org/fr/mdq/archives/00/2002/numero. aspx?num=2

Burstall, Dawn R.D., T. Micheal Vallis, Ph.D. and Geoffrey K. Turnbull, M. D., I.B.S. relief: A Doctor, a Dietitian and a Psychologist Provide a Team Approach to Managing Irritable Bowel Syndrome. Chronimed Publishing, Minneapolis, 1998. 176 p.

Canadian Society of Intestinal Research – SIR: www.badgut.com

Caron, André. 1995. *Le clinicien.* V. 10, n°s 10 and 11.

Chaire en gestion de la santé et de la sécurité du travail dans les organisations : Série La santé psychologique au travail... de la définition du problème aux solutions : http://cgsst.fsa.ulaval.ca :

T. 1 : *L'ampleur du problème - L'expression du stress au travail.*
T. 2 : *Les causes du problème - Les sources de stress au travail.*
T. 3 : *Faire cesser le problème - La prévention du stress au travail.*

Chang, Stephen T. 1984. *Le livre des exercices internes,* SIP, Stuyvesant Publishing Co.

Chaput, Marcel and Tony Lesauteur, 1971. Extracts of *Dossier Pollution,* Éditions du jour.

Collard, Christine. *Maladie de Crohn (MC) et recto-colite hémorragique (RCH).* In Quotipharm: http://www.quotipharm.com/Archives/Formation+Therapeutique-420/cette+semaine+Maladie+de+Crohn+et+RCH-222095.cfm

Corman, Louis : *Psychopathologie de la rivalité fraternelle,* Bruxelles 1970, Charles Dessart, Editor.

Côté, Jacinthe, Nutritionist, in *Le Soleil*, July 4th 2004, p. A-11; and in *Le Soleil*, January 23th 2005, page A-10.

Côté, Jacinthe, Nutritionist, *Une allergie qu'on appelle intolérance*, in *Le Soleil*, Mars 20th 2005, page A-13.

Crisafi, Daniel-J. ND. PhD. : *Candida albicans* : *Plusieurs ennuis de santé sont liés à cette levure - Fatigue, migraines, dépression, étourdissements*, Quebec 1994, FORMA.

Cyr, Josiane, Nutritionnist. In *Le Soleil*, May 20th 2000.

Dallaire, Christian D[r], *Helicobacter au pilori*, in *Le Clinicien – La revue de formation médicale continue*, STA communications Inc. Volume 1, February 1996, pp. 114 to 129.

de Compiègne, C.F. Mercier. *Éloge du pet, dissertation historique, anatomique et philosophique.* Apolline Edition - An VII de la Liberté, Paris, ISBN : 2-84556-016-8, 131 p.

de Cotret, Pierre René and Marie-Michèle Mantha. *La migraine. Passeport Santé* : http://www.passeportsante.net/fr/Maux/Problemes/Fiche.aspx?doc=migraine_pm

Dean, Carolyn, M.D., N.D., and L. Christine Wheeler, MA. IBS for Dummies. Wiley Publishing, Inc., Hobeken NJ, 2006. 362 p.

Dehin, Robert, Jocelyne Audry and Marie-Michèle Mantha. *L'insomnie. Passeport Santé* : http://www.passeportsante.net/fr/Maux/Problemes/Fiche.aspx?doc=insomnie_pm

Devroede, Ghislain. 2003. *Ce que les maux de ventre disent de notre passé*. Paris, Payot, 311 p.

Dextreit, Raymond. 1984. *Pour surmonter rapidement Spasmophilie et aussi Asthénie & Tétanie*. Paris, *Collection la santé dans ma poche, Éditions de la revue Vivre en harmonie*.

Dubé, Réjean. M. D. February 2002. *Le Médecin du Québec*, V. 37, No 2.: http://www.fmoq.org/fr/mdq/archives/00/2002/numero. aspx?num=2

Ducroux, Charles. Septembre 28th 2006. *Le Quotidien du pharmacien. Les insomnies.* N° 2428.: http://www.quotipharm.com/journal/index.cfm?dnews=122998&newsId=23&fuseaction=viewarticle&DArtIdx=376351

Dufour, Daniel. 2003. *Les tremblements intérieurs – Accepter de vivre ses émotions. Les Éditions de l'Homme.* 133 p.

D'Souza A.L. et collab. 2002. Probiotics in prevention of antibiotic associated diarrhea: meta-analysis. B.M.J., 324: 1361-4.

Eustache, Isabelle. M. D., in E-sante from an article of Renée D. Goodwin in Psychosomatic Medicine, November/December 2002. : http://www.e-sante.fr/ : http://www.e-sante.fr/francais/article.asp?idarticle=6753&idrubriq ue=189

Feldman, Catherine. M. D. In E-sante: http://www.e-sante.fr/francais/article.asp?idarticle=2031&idrubriq ue=57

Finley, Guy. *Lâcher prise, La clé de la transformation intérieure,* 1993 (1990), Le Jour Editor.

Guichard, Renaud. M. D., in E-sante: http://www.e-sante.fr/interview-faut-il-maigrir-tout-prix-avec-anneau-gastrique/actualite/838

Guide familial des symptômes, Éditions Santé et Éditions Fides, in Famili-Prix Inc. http://www.familiprix.com/savoirsante/ficheInformationSante/colon-irritable

Hachette, J.C. Dr; Lebert, N. : *Le guide de la médecine psychosomatique, comment guérir le corps en soignant l'esprit,* Paris, 1979, Marabout, 320p.

Hanauer, S. B. *Maladies inflammatoires de l'intestin.* In Nennett J.-C. et coll. *Cecil - Traité de médecine interne* – 1st ed. *Flammarion Médecine-Sciences*, Paris, 1997 : 707-715.

Haumont, Claude. *Le guide Marabout de la relaxation et de la sophrologie*, 1980, Verviers, *Les nouvelles éditions Marabout.*

Hébert, Isabelle. M. D. In *E-Sante* : http://www.e-sante.fr/

Howard, Nigel. *Comprendre le syndrome du côlon irritable*, Modus vivendi Inc. Montréal, 2003 142 p.

Jacobson, Edmond Dr, *Savoir relaxer pour combattre le stress*, 1980, Montréal, *Les Éditions de l'Homme.*

Jolicœur, Annie. Nutritionist. 2002. in *Du cœur au ventre*, AMGIF, 2, No. 1 Spring, pp. 2-3.

Kissel, P. et Barrucand, D. *Placebos et effet placebo en médecine*, Masson, Paris 1964.

Laforgue, René. M. D. : *Psychopathologie de l'échec*, Paris, *Petite Bibliothèque Payot.*

Lamontagne, Yves. M. D. : *Techniques de relaxation*, 1982, Montréal, *Éditions France-Amérique.*

Leberherr, Renaud. M. D. in E-sante: http://www.e-sante.net/

Ledoux, Stéphane M. D. *La migraine : ce qu'il faut garder en tête*, *Le Clinicien*, May 2004 p. 67-72. : http://www.stacommunications.com/journals/leclinicien/2004/May/PDF/067.pdf

Lemieux, Louis-Guy. in *Le Soleil*, January 23th 2005, page A-10.

Lehman, Stéphane M. D. *La migraine après 65 ans : ne pas faire n'importe quoi.* in E-Sante : http://www.e-sante.fr/francais/article.asp?idarticle=6176&idrubrique=25

Loiseau, Didier. M. D. *La diverticulose.* Erda Editions.

Lowen, Alexander. Dr. : *Le Corps bafoué*, 1976, *Éditions du Jour*.

Maher, Colette. *Rajeunir par la Technique Nadeau : Méthode de régénérescence*, 1984, *Les Éditions Québécor*.

Marcotte, Claude. *Vaincre la dépression par la volonté et l'action*, 1982, *Le Jour, Editor*.

Mayo Clinic, *Les maladies de l'appareil digestif.* 2000, Lavoie et Broquet. 244 p. : www.broquet.qc.ca

Médisite: Extracts from articles in: http://www.medisite.fr/

Montaigne (de), M. *Essais*. Tome I, *Livre premier,* chap. XXI. *Le livre de poche. Librairie générale française;* Paris 1972. In Lachaux, B. and Lemoine, P. *Placebo, un médicament qui cherche la vérité»*, Medsi/ McGraw-Hill, Paris 1988. : http://www.e-sante.fr/francais/article. asp?idarticle=17&idrubrique=54

Moriarty, Kieran J. *Comprendre le syndrome du côlon irritable, Médecine familiale, Les publications Modus Vivendi Inc.* From the original version : Understanding Irritable Bowel Syndrome, Family Doctor Publications 2000-2006. 132 p.: www.modusaventure. com

Northwestern Society of Intestinal Research: http://www.badgut. com

Oppenheim, Micheal. M. D., 1990. The Complete Book of Better Digestion – A Gut-Level Guide to Gastric Relief, Rodale Press Emmaus, Pennsylvania.

Pallardy, Pierre. *Et si ça venait du ventre? - Fatigue, prise de poids, cellulite, troubles sexuels, problèmes esthétiques, dépression, insomnie, mal de dos.* Robert Lafont, Paris, 2002, 257 p.

Paré, Pierre M. D., gastroenterologist and Marc Bradette M. D., gastroenterologist, *Les troubles digestifs fonctionnels* in *Le Clinicien*, Vol. 11, n° 4, April 1996.

Participate, International Foundation for Functional Gastrointestinal Disorders, Vol. 7, N° 2, Summer 1998, p 4-6 et Vol. 9, N° 4, Winter 2000. : http://www.iffgd.org/

Participate, International Foundation for Functional Gastrointestinal Disorders, Vol. 7, N° 2, Summer 1998, p 1-5 et Vol. 11, N° 1, Spring 2002. : http://www.iffgd.org/

Participate, International Foundation For Functional Gastrointestinal Disorders, Vol. 8, N° 1 Summer 1999. : http://www.iffgd.org/

Peck, M. Scott, M. D. People of the Lie, The Hope for Healing Human Evil, Touchstone Book, Simon & Schuster Publisher, New York, 1998. Or for the French version : *Les gens du mensonge*, 1983, *J'ai lu*, Paris.

Protégez-vous and PasseportSante.net Collection. 2006. *Guide des produits de santé naturels. Les Éditions Protégez-vous*, Montréal, 96 p. http://www.pv.qc.ca

Schiffman, Muriel. 1967. *Self Therapy: Techniques for Personal Growth, Self Therapy Press.*

Perreault, Danielle. M. D. 2004. In *Le Soleil*, March 28th, p. A-15.

Poitras, Pierre. M. D. gastroenterologist, in *Du cœur au ventre, Association du Syndrome de l'intestin irritable* (ASII) or *Association pour les maladies gastro-intestinales fonctionnelles* (AMGIF). : http://www.mauxdeventre.org

Poitras, Pierre. M. D. gastroenterologist, in *Du cœur au ventre*, AMGIF, Vol. 4, n° 4, Winter 2004.

Presles, Philippe. M. D. in E-sante: *Syncope vagale, rien de grave*, E-sante, October 8th 2002. from an article of Soteriade, New England Journal of Medicine, 347: 878-885, 2002. : http://www.e-sante.fr/francais/article.asp?idarticle=5985&idrubriq ue=214

Presles, Philippe. M. D. in E-sante : *Hémoroïdes : efficacité confirmée du Daflon*, E-sante, Octobre 13th 2004. :
http://www.e-sante.fr/magazine/article.asp?idArticle=7955&idRubrique=214&urldesc=A4H%c3%a9morro%c3%afdesefficacit%c3%a9confirm%c3%a9d

Presles, Philippe. M. D. *Yaourts et turista*, in E-sante, July 5th 2002. From an article of D'Souza A.L. et coll., Probiotics in prevention of antibiotic associated diarrhea: meta-analysis. B.M.J., 324: 1361-4, 2002. :
http://www.e-sante.fr/francais/article.asp?idarticle=5761&idrubrique=4

Presles, Phillippe. M. D. *L'origine bactérienne se confirme*, E-sante, October 6th 2004. From an article of Naser S.A. et coll., The Lancet, 364 : 1039-1044, 2004. :
http://www.e-sante.fr/maladie-crohn-origine-bacterienne-se-confirme/actualite/1084

Réal, Pierre. *Pour une vie heureuse... triomphez de l'angoisse*, 1963, Paris, Marabout Flash.

Rogé, Jacques. Pr, *Le mal de ventre*, *Éditions Odile Jacob*, Paris, 1998. 172 p. :
http://www.odilejacob.fr

Science, 297 : 2275-9, 2002. : http://www.sciencemag.org/

Servan-Schreiber, David. M. D. psychiatrist: *Guérir le stress, l'anxiété et la dépression sans médicaments ni psychanalyse*. Robert Laffont, Paris, 2003, 302 p.

Skrabaneck, P. et J. McCormick. Idées folles, idées fausses en médecine, Odile Jacob ed. Coll. Opus, Paris 1997, 196 p. : http://www.odilejacob.fr

The Inside Tract. *Intolerances.* In The Norhwestern Society of Intestinal Research, Diatary Management of Food Allergies. 1997. p. 191-3, In, n° 130, Mars-April 2002, p. 8-9.

Thompson, W. Grant M. D. Gut Reactions – Topics in Functional Gastrointestinal Disease: What are Placebos? Are they good for you? In *Participate*, 11, No. 4 Winter 2002, International Foundation for Functional Gastrointestinal Disorders IFFGD: http://www.iffgd. org

Tietze, G. : *Votre corps vous parle – écoutez-le*, Le Jour, editor, 1989, 211 p.

Tougas, G., Hwang, P., Paterson, W. G. and al. 1998 Dyspeptic symptoms in the general Canadian population: prevalence and impact on quality of life. Gastroenterology 114 (4 Pt 2) : A312.

Traitement des maladies inflammatoires de l'intestin. In « *GNP - Encyclopédie pratique du médicament 2000*. »; *Éditions du Vidal*, Paris 1999, 616-620.

Tulin, Michel. M.D. gastroenterologist. *Diarrhée et gastroentérite*, In E-sante, May 31st 2001 :
http://www.e-sante.fr/francais/article.asp?idarticle=1088&idrubriq ue=235&page=causes

Uexküll, von Thure. *La médecine psychosomatique*, 1996, Éditions Gallimard.

Viet-Quoc Nguyen, Patrick. B.A. Pharm. Québec Pharmacie, 51, no 7, pp. 572-576.

Wahnschaffe Gastroenterology 2001; 121: 1329-1338 and Sanders DS and coll. Lancet 2001; 358: 1504-8 in Egora: http://www.agora.fr

THE AUTHOR

Born in 1956 in Forestville on the North shore of the Saint-Laurence River, Quebec, Canada, the author has a bachelor degree in Philosophy (equivalence) from Laval University of Québec, Canada (1978), a bachelor degree in management economics (double honour) from Guelph University, Ontario, Canada (1984), and 30 credits at master level in economics from Laval University. He works for the government of Québec since 1986.

He has been initiated to transcendental meditation in 1980, to Nadeau technique en 1995, to Taï Chi in 2005 and to Qi Gong in 2008. He made psychoanalysis between 1988 and 1994; and he experienced many healing techniques (acupuncture, physiotherapy, phytotherapy, orthotherapy, chiropracy, and psychotherapy).

He suffers from dyspepsia and IBS since his birth. With the regular practice of his techniques, he passed from curing pain to prevent it. He is convinced that it is possible to **live a normal pain free life with functional gastrointestinal disorders.**

He published the first French version of this book in 1999. He wrote many articles on digestive track self-help in the *Journal Vert*, *Le Journal*, and in *Du Cœur au ventre*, the *Association des maladies gastro-intestinales fonctionelles* (AMGIF) review.